ANCIENT WISDOM
FOR WESTERNERS

ANCIENT WISDOM FOR WESTERNERS

A Short Introduction to Tibetan Medicine

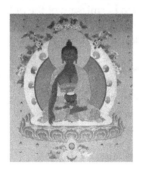

Marilyn Magazin

AEON

First published in 2022 by
Aeon Books

Copyright © 2022 by Marilyn Magazin

British Library Cataloguing in Publication Data

A C.I.P. for this book is available from the British Library

ISBN-13: 978-1-91350-496-0

Cover image: Medicine Buddha and Tibetan Plants from traditionalartofnepal.com
Illustrations by Phoebe Young

Typeset by Medlar Publishing Solutions Pvt Ltd, India

www.aeonbooks.co.uk

*I dedicate this book posthumously to
Geshe Lobsang Tengye, Jacques Haesaert and
Brigitte Jordan, who were my precious teachers,
therapists, and dear friends. I also dedicate this book
to Dr. Lobsang Shrestha, who continues to teach me.*

There is always something that can be done—
even if it's not the perfect solution.

TABLE OF CONTENTS

ACKNOWLEDGEMENTS xiii

PREFACE xv

INTRODUCTION xvii

Chapter 1

What is Tibetan medicine? 1

Chapter 2

Explanation of Buddhist concepts 9

Chapter 3

Anatomy, physiology, and psychology 17

Chapter 4

Conception, formation of the body, and childbirth 41

Chapter 5

What is health? 49

Chapter 6

Behavior and nutrition 51

Chapter 7

What is disease, disorder?..81

Chapter 8

Classes of diseases 83

Chapter 9

Invisible powers and spirits 85

Chapter 10

Symptoms and diagnosis...89

Chapter 11

What is healing? 99

Chapter 12

Therapy.. 101

Chapter 13

Western dogmas absent from Tibetan medicine.................... 117

Chapter 14

The Tibetan medicine approach to several common
      diseases 119

Chapter 15

Signs, omens, and dreams.. 129

Chapter 16

Astrology 131

CONCLUDING REMARKS.. 133

APPENDIX... 135

REFERENCES 143

SUGGESTED READING 145

INDEX... 147

ACKNOWLEDGEMENTS

Special thanks to my fellow members of the Association Ambroisie for their encouragement to use my personal learning experiences to write this introduction, and for their permission to include some figures from their book, *Introduction to Tibetan Medicine: Teachings of Jacque Haesaert*. I am also grateful to my sister, Pam O'Neil, and to Susan Peters who made many useful edits.

PREFACE

My work over a period of forty years as a research scientist and my interest in natural health incited my study with Tibetan medicine practitioners. I had the great fortune of discovering Tibetan Buddhism thirty years ago, at the Institut Vajra Yogini in France. In 1998, I began to study there with Jacques Haesaert (1942–2009), French naturopath and Tibetan medical doctor. He was taught by Dr. Ama Lobsang Dolma and Dr. Tsering Dinggang in India and then joined Mother Theresa's volunteers in Calcutta. After returning to Europe, Jacques Haesaert gave consultations and taught Tibetan medicine for more than thirty years in France and Spain. His wish was to bring together Tibetan medicine and Western medicine so their complementarity could be understood and utilized.

Jacques Haesaert and his students in France created Ambroisie, a non-profit association for the study and preservation of Buddhist Tibetan medicine, in 1991. After his passing, his students in France compiled an introduction to Tibetan medicine based on his teachings and notes. I have translated this book, *Tibetan Medicine—Medicine of Light: Teachings of Jacques Haesaert*, from French to English. His wish was to participate in the preservation of the authenticity and richness of this medical tradition, and the result is this comprehensive book with details of what he learned from his teachers and through his experience as a Tibetan doctor.

My intent here is to introduce readers, in a simple way, to this ancient wisdom, explaining why Tibetan medicine is so effective and suggesting ways to lead healthier and happier lives. I especially hope to incite the curiosity of Western physicians, for them to share what they learn from these pages with their own patients. Years of scientific investigation convinced me that the answers to many questions about the human body and disease can be found in traditional medicine systems.

Jacques Haesaert inspired me to remain in the spirit of the teachings, as he always did, rather than transmit literal teachings of Tibetan medicine that otherwise would have little value for most Westerners. This book will teach you of the origins of Tibetan medicine, and you will find some explanations of Tibetan Buddhist terms, as well as some specific advice that can directly benefit you. For this to be useful, one needs to be willing to make changes.

I have included some quotes and figures from *Tibetan Medicine—Medicine of Light, Teachings of Jacques Haesaert*. I have also included some specific information from translations of consultations and teachings by Dr. Lobsang Shrestha, with whom I continue to study Tibetan medicine.

INTRODUCTION

Tibet, a mystic land nested in the Himalayan mountains, remained isolated from the rest of the world for many centuries. Only recently has its medical system become the object of international interest, thanks to meetings between Western and Tibetan physicians and scientists, through the initiatives of the Dalai Lama. He has directed the effort to preserve the comprehensive healing tradition and all the other aspects of the rich Tibetan culture.

To understand the workings of Tibetan medicine, we need to open our minds to new concepts and notions, for we are entering into this world of intangible components that include invisible beings and spiritual practices. Probably the most striking difference between Western and Tibetan medicine that you will encounter is how Tibetan medicine looks at health and disease from an energetic perspective, as well from an anatomical and physiological one. It can be challenging for Westerners to understand and accept the notions of keeping these invisible subtle energies balanced and freely moving through invisible channels that are unquantifiable by scientific means.

It will become immediately clear that a Tibetan doctor treats the patient as a unique case and studies his condition globally. Rather than treating just the symptoms, a Tibetan doctor takes the patient's mental and emotional state, environment, and lifestyle into consideration. Age, family life, and working conditions are also pertinent factors, and special emphasis is put on behavior and food choices. Treatment always includes modification of the patient's nutrition and habits, to facilitate their needs at that particular time.

The good news is that we can start to apply effective preventive medicine and begin our own healing by taking into consideration our state and personal choices. We can reap the benefits of eliminating, or at least reducing, our actions that have negative repercussions on our health, both physically and emotionally. For example, Tibetan medicine explains that our physiological needs are not fulfilled by eating a lot of raw and cold foods and drinks in winter, when outdoor temperatures drop—we must adapt accordingly to the seasons. We could benefit from paying more attention to what our bodies are trying to tell us and avoid excessive consumption of sour foods and alcohol.

Explanations found in Tibetan medicine are based on logic, and centuries of experience has proven it to be effective. Discovering and addressing the causes for disorders explain the success of Tibetan treatments, especially of chronic disease. We shall see here the root causes of disease and what kind of changes can be made in order to reap substantial benefits.

I would like to stress from the offset that Tibetan doctors would not suggest that patients stop the treatment given by a Western doctor. There is a full understanding and appreciation of the benefits of modern medicine. The two systems are complementary! It is clear that Western medicine is well-equiped to treat emergencies and acute illness with the support of modern technology, such as scanners and precise surgical methodology. However, Tibetan medicine is particularly effective in treating long-standing disorders, such as arthritis, liver disease, poor blood circulation, as well as digestive disorders. It can also enhance the immune system and reduce inflammation. Success has been obtained in patients with asthma, eczema and depression, to name a few. Marked improvement can be obtained in patients with serious diseases, such as Parkinson and multiple sclerosis, and many cases of chronic disease. Although they cannot be cured, progression can be slowed down or eliminated; quality of life can be considerably improved.

It is not pleasant to be advised to do things differently in our lives, change our behavior and food choices, even give up aspects of our lives that we enjoy. Nevertheless, much of what follows is not that difficult to implement! The next step is to decide to apply what works for us. A Tibetan doctor would suggest that you take from their teachings what you find useful in order to have a healthy body and a happy state of mind.

I quote Jacques Haesaert: "Tibetan medicine is above all an art whose aim is to make men responsible for themselves, conscious of their potential for happiness, love and wisdom, and of the errors not to commit that which would lead them to suffering."

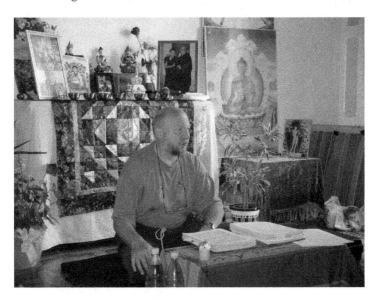

Figure 1A. Jacques Haesaert teaching in France.

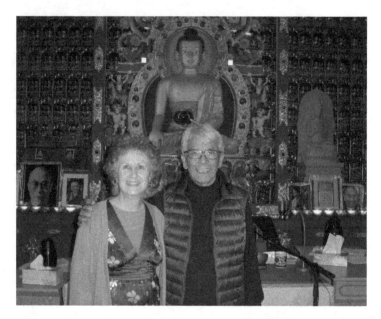

Figure 1B. Dr. Lobsang Shrestha with the author.

CHAPTER 1

What is Tibetan medicine?

First of all, the four fundamental aspects of Tibetan medicine are:

1. Providing relief from suffering, which is the vow of a physician, and doing this without discrimination, regardless of the patient's situation, whether they are rich or poor, humble or powerful.
2. Restoring the balance of the subtle energies and the corporal constituents, which are defined below.
3. Maintaining equilibrium.
4. Prolonging existence.

Tibetan medicine offers means of prevention, diagnosis, determining the causes of disease and suffering, treatment, and when death is near, comfort and preparation for the patient. A lot of this information could enrich Western medicine.

Tibetan medicine is an ancient and profound tradition, whose origins are based on the *Ambrosia Essence Tantra* (*Gyü Shi*, in Tibetan) taught by Buddha Shakyamuni. It is a four-part, 152-chapter medical text, dating from the 4th century A.D. It describes 84,000 kinds of suffering, the 404 principal disorders and the 1080 obstacles to good health, and their treatments.

This traditional medical system is above all a Buddhist medicine, which implies that it is governed by compassion and great morality. This love-compassion called *bodhicitta*, literally "enlightenment-mind", also includes the notion of charity. Spiritual practices are part of the healing process. However, it is not necessary to be a Buddhist to profit from such practices. It is said that just hearing healing prayers and *mantras* has great benefit for all. *Mantra* literally means "mind protection". They are sacred Sanskrit syllables that embody an aspect of spiritual power. Of course, prayers and practices according to other traditions are just as useful and Tibetan doctors would never suggest that one gives up one's own religion.

Tibetan medicine is a comprehensive holistic medical system, synthesizing the knowledge from many countries and traditions. Holistic medicine is the science of healing that considers the whole person: his body, mind, spirit, and emotions. Tibetan medicine has a long history, which has been passed down through the generations. A milestone was the initiative undertaken by Tibetan king Tri-Song, and later those by other kings, to synthesize important medical knowledge by bringing doctors and teachers from other traditions to Tibet, to live and exchange information, in order to enrich Tibetan medicine. Besides being a Buddhist science, it is, therefore, a synthesis of what is best in the ancient medical systems of Tibet, Nepal, Mongolia, China, India, Persia, and Greece. It is also influenced by the ancient Tibetan indigenous pre-Buddhist Bon culture, which emphasized the role of spirits in health and disease, and by the ancient Egyptian civilization. The result is a truly holistic approach to medicine, practiced since the 8th century. Tibetan medicine incorporated this knowledge in the spirit of Buddhism, treating other cultures and religions with great respect.

The teachings are focused on showing compassion and genuine interest for the patient's well-being, as well as extensive diagnostic techniques and treatments. Emphasis is placed on prevention and on taking responsibility for one's own health. The patient's attitude is, therefore, very important. Moreover, the key to health is inter-connectedness, with everything in nature, and balance, so the entire psycho-social environment of the patient is always taken into consideration.

Becoming a Tibetan doctor traditionally required twenty years of study. Education included learning a certain number of pages of medical and astrological texts by heart. Medical students have to learn the characteristics of all the medicinal plants traditionally employed, as well as the conditions of their harvesting, preparation, and storage. Teaching the *Gyü-shi* includes memorization of the Tibetan Medicine Tree, which is a representation of health and disease, their components, diagnoses, and remedies. The system is analogous to a tree consisting of three roots, nine trunks, forty-seven branches, 224 leaves, two flowers and three fruits, illustrated in Figures 2 to 4. All the components of the tree are listed in the appendix, in order to give the reader an idea of how detailed the information is. This tree is itself an introduction to Tibetan medicine. During the centuries of oral transmission of medical knowledge, it proved to be a priceless teaching tool.

The three-root system contains the body root, the diagnosis root, and the treatment root, which describe nutrition, behavior, medicines and other treatments. The tree (your body) can flourish only when the three life forces, also called the subtle energies, the seven bodily constituents, and the three excretory functions work in harmony.

Root one describes the general condition or state of a person, and it has two trunks. The first represents a healthy person in which body, energy, and mind are in a state of balance. The branches stand for general information and the leaves illustrate the details. The flowers represent health, purity, and brilliance/ longevity. The fruits represent dharma (the Buddha's teachings and doctrines), wealth, and happiness. The second trunk describes the types and causes of imbalance that result in disease.

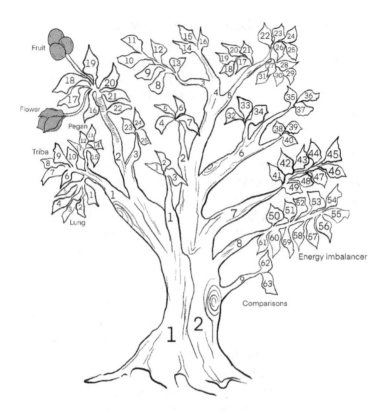

Figure 2. The medicine tree—root one.

Root two describes diagnostic techniques. The first trunk is that of observation of the patient's behavior and appearance. The first diagnostic technique is urinalysis. The second trunk describes touch diagnosis, with emphasis on the patient's pulses. The third trunk is questioning to understand the patient's case history, including their lifestyle, diet, emotional and physical states.

Root three describes methods of treatment, including therapeutic diet, modification of behavior, medication, and application of external therapies.

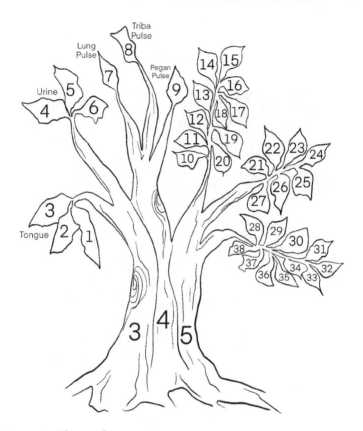

Figure 3. The medicine tree—root two.

A prime feature of Tibetan medicine is how the subtle energy level co-exists with the visible level of physical components in our body. These subtle energies govern everything that happens in our mind and body. Energy in this context refers to a dynamic power, considered to be the source of all existence.

For those hearing these explanations for the first time, they are, of course, as mind-boggling as explanations of parallel universes. We are talking about a system wherein three types

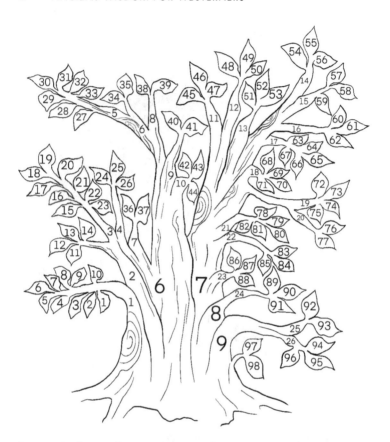

Figure 4. The medicine tree—root three.

of very subtle, therefore invisible, energies move through channels, controlling all bodily functions. This system explains the effects of acupuncture, shiatsu, Chi Gong, yoga, spiritual practices, phantom pain, spiritual healing, and many other unexplained healing processes. Moreover, here we find a logical explanation of the origins of mind and consciousness, as the physical presence of a brain alone is insufficient to comprehend the entirety of these aspects of ourselves.

Health, sickness, diagnosis, and treatment are explained in terms of balance of the three subtle energies: *lung, triba,* and *pegen*. I have chosen to use these terms transliterated in Jacques Haesaert's simple way, from Tibetan rather than the approximate translations: wind, fire, and phlegm, respectively, because they cannot be precisely translated into but a few words. These subtle energies will be explained in detail throughout this book.

Tibetan doctors have extensive knowledge of anatomy, physiology, embryology, and psychology. When patients are diagnosed and treated, many invisible factors are also taken into consideration. These include the three types of subtle energies, the chakras, subtle paternal and maternal "drops" or seeds, subtle channels, and spirits, none of which are accepted by Western science as they are unquantifiable by scientific means. Many components exist simultaneously on coarse, subtle, and very subtle levels.

Other major components of this medical system include the five elements (earth, air, fire, water, and space), which make up all physical substances; the cold or hot qualities of all substances, including foods, the importance of taste, behavior, timing, climate, spiritual practices, and astrology.

CHAPTER 2

Explanation of Buddhist concepts

B uddhism and Tibetan Medicine are intrinsically linked. In order to begin to understand the wisdom of Tibetan Medicine, it is necessary to gain some knowledge of Buddhist concepts. These include:

—**Mutual respect and confidence** in the doctor and in the treatments. Modern medicine sometimes considers some of the value we receive from this to be part of the "placebo effect." Tibetans consider this to be normal behavior when someone else is taking charge of your health.

—**Freedom from suffering and happiness as main goals in life.** Physical, mental, spiritual, and emotional sufferings are universal conditions of human life, and a lot of our time is spent trying to avoid or relieve them. Achieving these goals is possible, by altruism, which is the opposite of selfishness, and by appropriate attitude, thought and action, as explained in the following chapters.

—**Development of a kind heart and unbiased compassion for all living beings.** This is not pity but rather empathy, understanding, and respect. The moment that this is understood, real transformation can take place. We have all had the experience of feeling better after helping a person or an animal. We can experience far-reaching health benefits and eliminate a great deal of our own pain and suffering by turning our attention from our own problems toward those of others.

It is also important to have genuine compassion for ourselves, and do what we are capable of doing, according to our age, physical health, situation, and so on. A seventy-year-old person does not have the physical capacity of a twenty-year-old. We want to be kind to ourselves too! This will also help us develop greater self-esteem and satisfaction. Dissatisfaction is responsible for many disorders. Another aspect of maintaining good health is feeling gratitude to all who contribute to our well-being and for all the advantages we have, the people we have met and loved, opportunities, our material comfort, and the care we have received from others.

—The endless cycle of life, death, and rebirth, called *Samsara*. Buddhists believe in reincarnation, and explain that a being can be reborn in any one of the six "realms" of existence. What we think, we say, and we do determine our future. We thus create the *karma* to be reborn as a human or in another form. Right now, we are in the "human" realm, and it is said that this birth is extremely rare and precious. Only humans have the capacity to benefit from precious teachings and improve themselves. We are responsible for, and can take charge of, our health.

The six realms should also be understood as six ways to exist, and we ourselves create the energies of these planes. The energies are divided into six categories: pleasure and power for the realm of the *gods*, jealousy for the realm of the *demi-gods*, pride for the human realm, stupidity for the animal realm, avidity for the realms of the hungry ghosts (*pretas*, in Sanskrit), and evil for the hell realm. These realms are not really separate, and humans have contact with all of them, although they are usually only aware of humans and animals, since the other beings are invisible to us. We can experience each of these realms, as the darkest or the most heavenly, as they also represent the six states of mind that we can experience at any moment. Imagine the "hell" experienced at the loss of a child, or the physical suffering of dying in a fire. Imagine the endless joy of seeing your newborn baby.

The goal of a Buddhist is to become a progressively better person until finally all negativity is eliminated and he/she no longer needs to be reborn in *Samsara*. We can improve ourselves by contemplating and meditating, listening to qualified teachers, showing compassion for others, etc. It is a big step to finally understand that no one else is to blame for what happens to us. Of course, one does not have to be Buddhist or agree with the notions of rebirth or karma to understand the advantages eliminating blame on others for our misfortunes!

—The role of karma in health and disease. All our actions and thoughts can affect our health.

Jacques Haesaert quoted Lama Thubten Yeshe, his spiritual guide, who explained karma simply, as follows, "Karma is not something complicated or philosophical. Karma means watching your body, watching your mouth, and watching your mind. Trying to keep these three doors as pure as possible is the practice of karma."

Karma is a Sanskrit word, literally meaning "action". It is the law of cause and effect. Good karma is the fruit of virtuous actions that leads to happiness, and bad karma, which is the result of non-virtuous actions, leads to suffering. Our negativity also guides us to do more negative actions that will engender greater suffering. Nevertheless, this law of cause and effect is not one of reward or punishment, because it is governed by the force of universal love. Whatever occurs always comes according to our needs and our level of comprehension.

It is very important to understand that the karma that is accumulated by an action always depends on the person's motivation. For example, the negative karma resulting from a person killing someone is not the same if it is done out of jealousy and hatred, or if it is done in order to protect others from the "victim". In this case, we take on the negative karma of our action, however, the result is not that of great suffering because our motivation was pure.

We are never disconnected from everything around us, and this is why every action has an effect. Our body is the intermediary for the relationship between our mind and the external world. A person's whole life revolves around relationships, on coarse, subtle, and very subtle levels.

—The karmic connection between the physician and the patient. The quality of their relationship is important for the diagnostic and healing processes. Trust is especially important because it enables a doctor to help his patients. The karmic connection determines which people they are able to help, and the fact that a particular doctor cannot help everyone shows the importance of karma in these relationships and in healing, in general.

—The physician's high morality and motivation, which is never for money. Poor people are traditionally not expected to pay for treatment and the quality of life of the patient is always the concern of the physician. If the patient is incurable, the physician should not give them curative treatments, even if they risk their reputation and loss of patients' confidence for chosing not to continue treatment. This would be uselessly prolonging or increasing the patient's suffering.

—Mindfulness: being conscious of whatever we are doing, being in the moment instead of projecting ourselves into the future or living in the past. When we eat, it is best to just eat, without other activities or distractions. The food is better assimilated and appreciated. Even a mundane act like washing dishes can be looked upon as something agreeable, because of its contribution to our good health and that of our family and friends! Being fully conscious of what we are doing can also help us get all the benefits from it and avoid committing errors. We can spend our time on what is essential in life, instead of trivial undertakings.

Being mindful is also helpful for those assisting the patient. It facilitates perception and understanding of the patient's needs, allowing us to find things that can be done to increase their comfort and reduce their suffering.

—Impermanence; for nothing is permanent no matter how much we wish it were. Relationships change, people leave us, we lose possessions, our youth, even eventually our lives, so appreciate here and now who we are and what we have! Unpleasant occurrences are also impermanent; knowing that suffering ends in one way or another is also a big consolation. Understanding that everything is impermanent includes accepting change and death, so the fear of them will not become even worse than their happening. Some patients who are full of fear say that not knowing what disease they had was worse than getting news that their condition was very serious. The doctor is honest with the patient.

We have all met people who give off a feeling of well-being and kindness, while others repel people around them and make others feel uncomfortable. Our perception is on a subtle energetic level, as well as the physical level of their actions, and explanations can be found, once we understand the workings of the subtle energies and karma. Meanwhile, it can be useful to think about impermanence when we are obliged to pass time in the presence of a "disagreeable" person. We can reflect on the fact that at this moment, the person is perceived as offensive or even as an enemy but awareness of impermanence allows us to realize that sometime in the future, this individual may even become our friend. Buddhists go farther, meditating on the fact that in some future life, the person may even be our mother. Thinking in this way, we can change our attitude drastically and live more peacefully.

—Consciousness creates the body. In the heart of Buddhism lies the belief that the consciousness of each of us is eternal, going from life to life in cycles of rebirth, and that it is this consciousness that is the very essence of us that creates the body. Tibetan medicine also teaches that our mind creates our happiness and good health, as well as our suffering and disease. Western medicine readily accepts the reality of patients experiencing psychosomatic disorders, so it is really not much of a leap to understand how Buddhists embrace the concept that mind creates the body and determines what happens to it.

—The root causes of all suffering and disease are "the three mental poisons". This is a basic principle of Buddhism and Tibetan medicine. These three poisons are 1) ignorance 2) desire, and 3) hatred/anger.

Ignorance means not understanding how things really exist—i.e., how all things are empty of intrinsic existence and nature, and "exist" because our mind gives them labels. This is what is meant by the Buddhist concept of emptiness. Thanissaro Bhikkhu explains this very well in his article in Tricycle published in1997, *What Do Buddhists Mean When They Talk About Emptiness?* Here, "desire" means uncontrolled desire and dissatisfaction.

These poisons destroy our happiness and cause disorders by disrupting the balance of the three subtle energies, *lung*, *pegen*, and *triba*, which are the links between these poisons and disease. These energies are responsible for the formation of the body and all its functions. Contributing causes and conditions also affect the subtle energies and determine whether we will get sick or not. Health and disease are, therefore, explained on a subtle energetic level and on mental and emotional levels, as well as on the physical.

—**A person is made up of "the five aggregates"**, which are form, sensation, perception, mental formations, and consciousness. All five must be present for any person to exist. This is a concept that goes beyond considering that a person consists of a body and a mind.

—**The person's "vital force" is eventually used up, resulting in death.** Certain behavior uses up this vital force, or vital energy (*La*, in Tibetan) more quickly, resulting in earlier death. There are spiritual practices that can be undertaken to increase one's vital force. *La* is the person's aura and its color is a function of the person's vital energy. We know the aura as the feeling or the quality that is perceived as surrounding or radiating from someone.

CHAPTER 3

Anatomy, physiology, and psychology

These subjects were explained in great detail in the *Gyü Shi*, centuries before much information was known in the West. The vocabulary used in the texts can thus appear strange to Westerners, and the centuries-old medical drawings may appear simple or naive. This does not mean that Tibetan physicians know little about anatomy and physiology. In fact, Tibetan medicine developed detailed knowledge of these subjects through dissection. Moreover, it was common practice to dissect the body of the deceased. The country's harsh terrain and climate and lack of wood for cremation made it necessary to practice sky burials, which consist of cutting up bodies and feeding them to vultures, in the presence of the family.

Tibetan medicine also explains a lot about what is unknown in modern anatomy and physiology, providing information that complements rather than contradicts Western medicine. The workings of the subtle energetic system that governs all bodily functions explain many phenomena that have remained unanswered. It is a kind of "missing link" between the mental and the physical, the mind and the body, and provides logical reasoning for why disease recurs, which is that the root cause was not removed. There are also complementary explanations for why some people fall ill in the presence of pathogens while others do not, and why some heal and others not, under the same circumstances and with the same treatment.

Elements of anatomy include the corporal constituents, the vital points, the circulatory system, and the body's openings, which are entry points. The corporal constituents are: 1) chyle produced from food; 2) blood, which humidifies the body and maintains life; 3) flesh, which covers the body; 4) fat, which lubricates it; 5) bone, the body's support; 6) marrow, the essential nutrient and 7) regenerative fluid, which is responsible for conception. There are coarse, subtle, and very subtle corporal constituents.

The vital points are specific places in the body that must remain intact in order for life to continue. These points are classified into seven types: those of flesh, fat, bone, ligaments, vessels, and the two types of organs, called solid organs and hollow organs.

Physiology covers the workings of the physical components of the body, which are the objects of disease and the subtle energies, which cause disease. As we shall see below, the correct functioning of the digestive system plays a crucial role in maintaining health and its correct functioning is always taken into account when treating disease. The three subtle energies must be balanced in order to maintain good digestion and assimilation of nutrients. Too much or too little of any of the three energies causes disorders.

Rhythms are divided into internal rhythms, innate in man that can be controlled to a certain extent, and external rhythms, that cannot. Examples of rhythms are inhalation/exhalation, cardiac rhythm, and circadian rhythms (wake/sleep cycles). Life is impossible without movement. Moreover, without the dynamic interplay of the female and male energies, beings could not exist, as there would be no manifestation. The red female energy is the energy of manifestation and externalization; the white male energy is reintegration and the tendency towards rest. Everything is born through the union between the "means or method" of the male energy and the "wisdom" of the female energy. The loss of one of the two energies inevitably leads to death. It should be noted that in the Himalayan tradition of Buddhism, the male quality is lunar, while the female quality is solar, which is the reverse of the Hindu tantric traditions.

Tibetans define all substances and processes in terms of the five elements: earth, air, water, fire, and space. They make up all matter of both the body and the external world to which a person's consciousness must connect in order to experience sensations. The seven corporal constituents are composed of the five elements, and each element has particular importance for one or more of these constituents. Earth, associated with the color yellow, predominates in bones and in marrow; water, associated with the color green predominates in lymph and blood; fire, associated with the color red, predominates in blood; and air, associated with white, predominates in all of them without dominating any of them. Space is associated with the color blue and is also necessary for the body to function.

Understanding the relationships between the five elements is important. The quantity of each element in relation to the others, along with the taste and the hot or cold quality of food determines which nutrients can be used as treatment, to pacify an excess or deficiency of one of the three subtle energies.

The three mental poisons

In order to understand how the three subtle energies function, we must first establish an understanding of the Buddhist concept of the three mental poisons—the primary causes of all our suffering and disease. They are not themselves "energies", but are rather the seeds created by our minds. As we have seen, the three are translated as ignorance, desire/attachment, and hatred/anger.

They are concepts that are not easy to understand, and can only be approximately explained in a few paragraphs.

Ignorance has nothing to do with formal education and acquiring facts and competence. It is a "wrong" view of how things exist. It would take a separate book to explain it clearly, but it is useful to have an idea of what this means. First, we need to understand what is conventional truth and ultimate truth. At the level of conventional truth, which is the way we normally see things, there is separation and discrimination between us and all that surrounds us. We think we exist as an independent being.

Conventional truth says "I" exists. However, ultimately, "I" is only fulfilling this definition of the word we consensually use for this object (my body and my mind). We can try to find and identify it, by asking; "Am I my arms or heart, or my face, my emotions, or my ability to talk, or is "I" just a word we have given to the collection of all the components that must have come from somewhere?"

As Lama Thubten Zopa Rinpoche explains, "What you see, what you hear, what you think, what you taste, what you touch—all the objects—are merely labeled by your mind."

Unlike conventional truth, ultimate truth means that nothing exists on its own as a single entity or object. Everything is dependent on everything else. A body and a mind are not sufficient for me to have existence. My body could not exist if it were not for my mother and father. This line of thinking can be extended to the fact that I would not exist if it were not for all the persons and things needed for my survival: the persons who gave me access to essential things, and the persons who gave birth to those persons, components like food, the sun, and water enabling the plants that provide food to grow, and we could continue indefinitely along these lines, for everything is interconnected.

In the realm of the ultimate, everything is in everything else.

Ignorance prevents us from understanding that the notion of independent existence is the cause of our suffering. Ego is separation from our surroundings and from other beings. and it creates in us three types of sentiments: I like, I don't like, and I'm indifferent. Ignorance obscures our view so we see only the negative side of our "enemy" and do not look at him from all angles, in order to discover his positive aspects.

It is clear that the three poisons distort our perception as to where suffering is coming from and what it means to be truly happy.

Desire is a poison, though this does not mean that we must rid ourselves of all desires. Chocolate and sex can bring us happiness, although not the lasting satisfaction, like that of saving a life or even having helped someone in need. Being satisfied is key to good health. The poison of desire means wanting to possess or control a person or an object, which can lead to disappointment and jealousy that prevent us from truly experiencing any happiness. Dissatisfaction leads to frustration and to then to disease, for no other person nor any possessions can be responsible for our happiness.

Moreover, we can never possess another being. We cannot even own an object indefinitely. Everything is impermanent and our favorite shoes or our most comfortable chair will get old too. Many persons in love consider that their lover should make them happy. Jacques Haesaert liked to quote Lama Thubten Yeshe, who compared this to our precious morning cup of coffee. "If we can have it the way we like it, then we are happy, but if one time if it does not taste right, we may become unhappy or even angry." Extrapolated to our lover, we can quickly become upset with him/her if this person's actions do not match our desires and expectations. Our partner or anyone else cannot be responsible for our happiness."

Our happiness can be easily destroyed by small irritations in life, leading to sleeping problems and even depression.

We cannot prevent unpleasant things from happening, but we can change our way of looking at the situation and our way of thinking. As we develop love as a virtuous state of mind, we want our loved ones to be happy, even if this means the end of our relationship or a separation with someone to whom we have become attached.

When the person we love leaves us, we think the pain is coming from our love for him/her, but love is not the cause of our suffering. Love is never the cause; the cause is attachment. Attachment is like a vampire living in us, creating needs and expectations, and even self-pity. Some persons become consumed by jealousy and suffer more from the jealousy than from the loss of their loved one. They feel genuine physical suffering. Doesn't it make more sense to develop compassion for ourselves, instead?

Once we have understood that it is worth doing the work on ourselves to eliminate, or at least reduce these "mental poisons", we can reap the benefit. When a situation arises, if there is something that can be done to resolve the problem, then it is worth doing it, but if not, then it is better to just let it go. Again, an example is to accept that a person has left you for another, and move on. Our jealousy serves no purpose. It does not even give the "satisfaction" of revenge because it does not punish those who hurt us. It only punishes ourselves. If someone else has obtained the promotion or the very thing that we desired, by trying to be happy for that person and generating positive thoughts toward them, we can transform our minds!

A person full of **anger and hatred** will lead a miserable life and eventually destroy their own health. This type of personality may eventually develop a disorder of the heart or liver. We all know that episodes of anger make us feel physically unwell, with a reddened face and a rapid heartbeat. Under the control of anger, we may hurt the very beings who are the dearest to us. Our egos are truly diabolical, sometimes inflicting verbal wounds that are even more painful than any physical hurt.

On the other hand, legitimate anger should arise in us against our ego. In this way, the energy of anger can be used to destroy the power our ego has over us.

I cite a personal experience:

One day at work, my director with whom I had a good relationship, came to see me and was visibly upset. He held a piece of paper up to me and said with anger, almost shouting, "Marilyn, you changed your recuperation day AGAIN and I'm fed up. You have done it again and again. I'm not going to sign it." I knew I would not succeed in getting a word in, so I remained silent. Facing such a surprising reaction, he puffed and went away. A couple of colleagues came to me, after hearing the scene. "Wow, what was that? He was so aggressive and you didn't say anything". I explained to them that anyway, it would have only fueled an argument, so I remained silent. They thought I should have responded. I told them that his anger surely had nothing to do with me and was probably set off by some other event, so I put up my virtual mirror and did not *take* what he was giving me. I took on none of his negativity, but rather, it just reflected it back to him. Why should I get upset for such a small thing? Then I went back to my office, for I was sure he would come and apologize in a few minutes. And sure enough, he came soon and tapped on the door. I smiled and said, "Things are better now?". He shyly smiled and handed me the signed (approved) form and started to apologize but I just added, "In fact, I changed the date because Dr. B and Dr. F. (my two Parisian collaborators) called me to say they are coming Friday". He smiled and went out. There was no reason for melodrama and NO hard feelings. I had learned to recognize that *he* had been having a bad day and his anger had nothing to do with me.

We don't openly greet unwanted guests who come into our houses, but we accept feelings of anger and hatred as "normal" and nourish them. We can learn to look at these emotions as they arise and decide to not accept them. We can let them go, instead of hanging on to them. As we start to understand that our negative emotions destroy our peace of mind, even our happiness, we realize that it is worthwhile to try to take control before disorder and disease manifest, because each of these three poisons increases one of the subtle energies and the resulting imbalance translates into disease.

Ringu Tulku, in his book, *Daring Steps: Traversing the Path of the Buddha* states, "When, for instance, strong anger or desire arises, a Vajrayāna* practitioner is not afraid of it. Instead, he or she would follow advice along the following lines: Have the courage to expose yourself to your emotions. Do not reject or suppress them, but do not follow them either. Just look your emotion directly in the eye and then try to relax within the very emotion itself. There is no confrontation involved. You don't do anything. Remaining detached, you are neither carried away by emotion nor do you reject it as something negative. Then, you can look at your emotions almost casually and be rather amused."

*N.B. Vajrayāna is a form of Buddhism, also called tantric Buddhism. In Tibetan Buddhism, the term tantra refers to various texts and the systems of meditation of the tradition.

Working to control and eventually eliminate negative emotions is a main feature of Buddhism and Tibetan medicine. Fortunately, there are many exercises and practices that can be done on our level to better understand the object of our negativity, diminish our ignorance, anger, and excessive desire, develop compassion even for those who harm us, and transform our minds. These include listening to teachings by qualified teachers, spiritual practices, developing compassion, and meditation. These methods and others, such as yoga, Tai Chi Chuan, and Chi Gong, provide the help we need. More and more medical studies are convincing Western doctors of this. For example, the benefits of meditation have been clearly proven in scientific studies of its effects on patients with high blood pressure, diabetes, stress, arthritis, and migraine.

So, how do we go from negative emotion to disease?

Emotions affect the three subtle energies, and the resulting imbalances cause the disorder when contributing causes and conditions are also present. When the three subtle energies are balanced and in their correct positions in the body, the person remains healthy. With an excess or deficiency of one or more of these subtle energies, the body cannot function properly and remains unhealthy until equilibrium is re-established. Many other subtle components are acting here and even their functioning does not explain everything that is going on. We shall see some examples later.

What is happening is, thus, not only on a visible biochemical and physiological level. Of course, hormones, neurotransmitters, and other components are involved, as Candace Pert elegantly explains in her book, *Molecules of Emotions: The Science Behind Mind-Body Medicine*.

Explanation of the three subtle energies

Health and disease are always explained in terms of cold and hot energy and in terms of balance of the three subtle energies, *body constituents, and waste products*. Of these, energy is the most important, for it is the vital link between body and mind. These subtle energies, which are also called the "internal vital principles" or "humors", are called *lung, triba* and *pegen,* in Tibetan. They are equivalent to the Ayurveda *doshas: vata, pitta*, and *kapha*. An accurate translation from Tibetan is impossible since these concepts are largely unknown in the West. Therefore, throughout this book, the terms transliterated from Tibetan are used. Subtle energies are also described in Chinese and Japanese medicine.

The energy formed by and affected by ignorance is *pegen*. The energy created by desire is *lung*, and the energy created by hatred is *triba*.

Characteristics of the three subtle energies are summarized below.

THE THREE SUBTLE ENERGIES

MENTAL "POISONS"		SUBTLE ENERGIES
DESIRE/ **ATTACHMENT/** **DISSATISFACTION**	creates >	*LUNG:* Ayurvedic *Vata* *"Wind"*
		• Air and space elements • Movements in the body • Neutral, light, thin, dry • Intelligence and memory • Mental afflictions
ANGER/HATRED	creates >	*TRIBA:* Ayurvedic *Pitta* *"Bile"*
		• Fire and space elements • Color, brilliance, force • digestion, body temperature • Liver, gall bladder, • Skin disorders
IGNORANCE	creates >	*PEGEN:* Ayurvedic *Kapha* *"Phlegm"*
		• Water, earth, space elements • Stability, structure • Cold, heavy, slow • Creamy, oily, thick • Body fluids

Where do these subtle energies come from?

Buddhists explain that the very subtle energy, *sokzin lung*, the energy that sustains life, creates the other very subtle energies, in response to one's desire for existence. *Sokzin lung* continues, from life to life, each time leading the consciousness, which left a previous incarnation, to the new incarnation so that the new body will come into existence at the moment of the union of the sperm and the ovum. In order to connect to the world of the five elements, and thus form its body, the consciousness must create specific "connective" energies from *sokzin lung*. Next, other subtle *lung* energies, each associated with an element, are then created. During the whole developmental process, all the other subtle energies arise in a specific order, as they are needed.

All physiological functions are controlled by the three energies

Lung **energy** governs all movements and other actions in the body and is associated with the element air and the neutral quality. It controls inhalation and exhalation, and expels substances, such as saliva and urine. This subtle energy moves through the components of the body, which are the objects of illness. Passing through the blood vessels, it keeps them clear of impurities. *Lung* is responsible for both intelligence and memory. It also affects the other two subtle energies, with the characteristic of increasing the heat of *triba* and the cold of *pegen* by "blowing" on these energies, just as wind makes a fire more intense. This is the reason why balanced *lung* is essential for the other two energies.

There are five types of *lung:*

Sokzin lung (life supporting) is the vital *lung* that goes from life to life. It is also responsible for breathing, swallowing food, sneezing, clearing the senses and intellect, and keeping the mind steady.

Kyengyu lung (ascendant) controls speech, increases the vigor of the body, and promotes mental endeavors.

Kyabche lung (omnipenetrating) controls walking, stretching, lifting objects, movements of the mouth, eyelids, anus, etc.

Menyam lung (metabolic) promotes digestion and metabolism.

Thursel lung (descendent) expels excrement, urine, semen, and menstrual blood and pushes the baby out at the time of birth.

Triba **energy** is responsible for metabolism and is associated with the fire element and is hot in quality. It is, therefore, "energy" itself. Its nature is hot, but this heat can be decreased by an excess of *pegen* or by a lack of *lung*. *Triba* is associated with bile and blood, is responsible for hunger and thirst, and makes digestion and absorption of nutrients possible. It increases body heat, gives courage, color to the body, confidence, and the power to accomplish our desires.

There are five types of *triba:*

Juche triba (digestive) controls digestion, the breaking down of essential nutrients, and then the separation of essence from waste.

Danggyur triba (color-transforming) is the driving force for achievement. *Drubche triba* (accomplishing) is responsible for the red color of essential nutrients in blood.

Thongche triba (visually-operating) controls vision.

Doksel triba (complexion-clearing) clears the skin and gives it a healthy color.

Pegen **energy** controls fluids in the body and is associated with the water and earth elements and is cold in quality. It keeps the mind and body firm, enables sleep, and lubricates the whole body, maintaining humidity in joints and keeping the skin soft. It is responsible for patience and mental and physical adaptation to external situations, such as a change in the outside temperature. *Pegen* is associated with an excess of phlegm and with bodily fluids. Its nature is cold but can become hot if associated with *triba*.

There are five types of *pegen:*

Tenche pegen (supporting) supports the other four *pegen* and the earth and water elements in the body.
Nyagche pegen (mixing) is responsible for mixing solid food with liquids into a semi-solid state.
Nyongche pegen (experiencing) controls the experience of taste.
Chorche pegen (connecting) is responsible for joint flexibility.
Tshimche pegen (satisfying) increases and satisfies the five senses.

Each of these subtle energies has its correct position in the body and must not go to other regions, otherwise disorders develop. The normal position and movement of these principal lung, triba and pegen energies are illustrated in Figure 5.

Everything that happens in our bodies is the result of movement and action of these subtle energies: when our food is digested, a muscle stretched, a wound healed, or a songbird heard. To better understand the ways that these energies function, try to get a feeling, for example, of how fits of anger are characterized by a *triba* excess; how obesity and slow movement are associated with excess *pegen*; and dry skin or diarrhea are associated with excess *lung* energy. The texts also refer to a fourth type of energy, called *blood*, which is related to blood but not limited to it. It has certain characteristics of *triba* but also has some different characteristics.

Jacques Haesaert explained that "for the energies to be balanced, our relations with the exterior must also be balanced, by acting with wisdom, love, compassion, and tolerance or renunciation, which are the opposites of the energies of ignorance, hatred, anger, and excessive sexual desire."

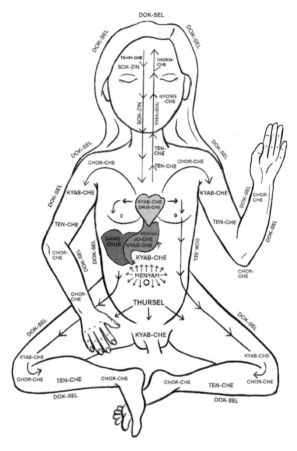

Figure 5. The subtle energies and their principal paths.

A person's dominant energy type

Everyone has a dominance of one of the types of subtle energy, which can be determined by the doctor, by observation of physical features, behavior, reading of the pulse, and other methods. In order to make a correct diagnosis and treat the patient, and give advice about the best foods to eat and which to avoid, it is important for the physician to know which subtle energy is dominant. Observation includes that of the patient's facial features, body shape, form, and height. A person's heredity is partially responsible for these characteristics, which give their predispositions and tendencies. Categorizing patients helps the doctor determine which types of medicines are best adapted to the person's constitution, personality, and character. It is also possible to deduce their strengths and weaknesses. This information can be wisely used in a child's early years, to help them use their strengths appropriately and overcome the weaknesses.

The following describes characteristics influenced by the dominant energies:

People influenced predominantly by *lung* often have angular features and a tendency to be bent over, with dry skin and a dark complexion. Their bones and articulations may protrude. They are generally small and thin, talkative, and often agitated. These people often feel cold. They prefer sweet, sour, and spicy foods. In addition, they generally have few possessions.

The situation is quite different for a person with a *lung* deficiency, who has a tendency to be inactive, sad, indecisive, with little desire to do anything. They may have a tendency to concentrate on the difficultly of things and be conformist and narrow-minded.

A person with a normal quantity of *lung* is open-minded, flexible, and respectful of others. They have intelligence and the ability to concentrate and persevere.

People influenced by a predominance of *triba* are often hungry and thirsty. They perspire abundantly and may give off a strong odor. Their complexion and hair are often yellowish, corresponding to their biliary character. They are of average height and are often proud, with sharp minds. They like sweet, bitter, and refreshing food.

A person with *triba* deficiency is the opposite, with a short trunk, compared to his legs and head. They lack self-esteem, so may even have little respect for themselves or others. This type of individual has a tendency toward laziness, imagining projects without ever completing them, and a lack of generosity.

When *triba* is balanced, the person's mind and actions are too. They are honest, respectful, compassionate, humble, patient, with the will to realize projects.

Persons with a predominance of *pegen* have large, heavy, roundish bodies and a tendency towards obesity. A baby's large head is characteristic of the *pegen* type. These persons generally have a light complexion, good posture, and adapt well to mental challenges. They sleep a lot, are peaceful and of a kind nature and do not anger easily. Their food preferences are spicy, sour, thick, and rough food.

When a person has *pegen* deficiency, they may suffer from a lack of fluids.

A person with balanced *pegen* is easy-going and adaptable.

Dominance of a particular energy depends on many factors. Each of the three energies has an association with our different stages of life/age. *Lung* is the dominant energy of the elderly. *Pegen* energy, and the water element that is associated with it, decrease as a person ages, so there is loss of muscle mass and a decline in mental faculties. The elderly have a tendency to have dry skin. Children, whose dominant energy is *pegen* sleep a lot, whereas the elderly generally sleep much less.

As we shall see below, seasonal influences, altitude, climate, and weather affect the three energies in different ways. As a result, disorders of the three energies are more likely to arise during specific times of the year. Changes in food choice and behavior are, therefore, important, regardless of the person's dominant energy.

Other elements of anatomy and physiology

In order for subtle energies and substances to circulate throughout the body, other components are needed; **the channels** (*tsa*, in Tibetan). The circulatory system consists of all the thousands of vessels that transport air, blood, bile, and lymph around the body. Some of these channels have openings through which the impurities exit, assure the functioning of the nervous system, and circulate the subtle energies. Some channels are coarse and others are subtle, therefore, invisible. The most subtle channels are the pathways of the subtle energies.

Invisible channels enable the energies carrying the most subtle male and female *drops* or *essences* (*thig-le*, in Tibetan) and sensations to circulate. This system consists of a central channel and right and left channels of the body that are connected to the 72,000 minor coarse vessels and the 12,000 subtle vessels. The middle, central channel is associated with *lung* energy and the nervous system. There is a connection between it and the spinal column, but they are not the same. The right channel is associated with *triba* and blood circulation and is hot in nature. The left channel is associated with *pegen* energy and the lymphatic and endocrine systems and is cold in nature.

When the internal passageways are damaged, accidentally or by poor nutrition or inappropriate behavior, the resulting blockages disturb movement of the three energies and disorders arise.

Specific *lung* energies control the opening and closing of passageways. For example, in the case of diarrhea, the rectal passageway does not close normally and in the case of constipation, it does not open sufficiently, due to a *lung* disturbance, which, of course, is not entirely responsible for these disorders. Here again, we have visible and invisible components acting together.

Channels converge at focal points, called **chakras** or *energy* centres, which take the form of a wheel. Each of these chakras has a particular role on the psychic, physical, and spiritual levels and possesses a particular quality. In the Tibetan medical system, there are five principal chakras, shown in Figure 6, and there exist many others. Each of the five chakras is associated with one of the five *lung*, a color, and represents a specific characteristic of the Buddha. The crown chakra (white) is associated with life-supporting *lung* and wisdom; the throat chakra (red), with ascendent *lung* and satisfaction; the heart chakra (blue), with pervasive *lung* and compassion; the navel chakra (yellow), with metabolic *lung* and generosity; and the genital chakra (green), with descendant *lung* and patience. Color therapy, as known in the West, is acting at the level of the chakras, as well as on a visual and an emotional level. The specific qualities of Buddha are antidotes for the emotions of ignorance, desire, anger, pride, and jealousy, respectively. Our ego is the root of all of them.

CHAKRA

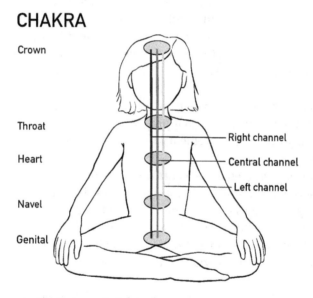

Figure 6. Chakras and channels.

The whole process of conception and formation of the body is described in great detail in the medical texts. Certain vital elements that explain how a new life can begin are unknown in Western science and medicine. These include **the white and red drops** (*thig-le*), which are the paternal and maternal *seeds* or *essence* that exist on the most subtle level to the coarsest. During a person's life, the two most subtle drops remain joined in the center of the heart and then spread throughout the body in less subtle forms. On a coarser level, the drops are the semen, which corresponds to the coarse white drop and the ovum, which corresponds to the coarse red drop. All body components are formed from the drops and the five elements.

Tibetans explain that conception is dependent on the law of karmic attraction between the parents and the incarnating consciousness. At the moment of conception, the individual's consciousness carried by *sokzin lung* enters the unified *drops* (the fertilized egg), which is the first external element of the incarnating being. The whole form of the new body is inscribed in them. The contributions from the mother and father and past generations to the new being thus exist in subtle and coarse forms.

Although Buddhists accept that parents make conception and birth possible, the mother and father are not considered to have caused the new existence to come about. Western science tells us that the brain develops in the new body, which in turn is responsible for sensory, motor, and mental functions. Here, we see that the child's body does not create its own consciousness because it existed even before conception!

Another big difference between Tibetan medical teachings and modern physiology concerns the digestive system, and the components of physiology as explained in Tibetan medicine challenges the Western mindset. Therefore, in order to better picture how the three subtle energies act, here is a simplified explanation of how they direct the process of eating and digestion:

A person puts a spoonful of food in their mouth and immediately the three subtle energies come into play. *Lung* energy guides the movements of the mouth, the tongue, and the food, so it can be chewed into small pieces and mixed with the liquid of *pegen*, and the *triba* energy of enzymes in saliva, such as amylase and lysozyme, to begin the digestion process. *Lung* moves the pieces through the esophagus as more *pegen* energy moistens them further. In the stomach, the three subtle energies act in coordination to secrete digestive enzymes. *Pegen* maintains the necessary moisture and coolness so the "digestive fire" of *triba* can further break down the food, without destroying the walls of the stomach. The transforming products move down through the digestive tract and the liver enables further transformation, separation, and assimilation of the final products, before they are finally eliminated as waste in the form of urine and faeces.

The processes of digestion, transformation of food, and separation into what is used and what is eliminated are referred to as *the seven extractions*, which are explained with regard to the three subtle energies.

The body metabolises nutrients into an essence that feeds and forms the "seven bodily constituents": nutritional essence (the essential nutrients from ingested foodstuffs), blood, flesh, fat, bone, marrow, and regenerative fluid. All the constituents constantly interact with each other. The three excretory functions: urine, excrement, and perspiration play vital roles and are not only considered as waste products. Solid waste in the intestines and urine in the bladder sustain the organs, as well as the substances situated above them. They keep the digestive products in place so they can be processed. Only then are the impurities expelled. Perspiration keeps the skin flexible and provides protection from the entrance of undesirable substances through the pores. Excretions are also important for diagnosis, providing the doctor with precious information.

The ultimate product of the seven extractions is *dang*, which is essence, light, *prana*. It takes seven days from the time food is ingested to the production of *dang*. If the energies are not balanced or if there is an excess of cold or hot energy in the organs, the corporeal constituents are not correctly made and the *dang* is of poor quality; liquids accumulate because the passageways of the body are closed. If one of the energies is too weak, digestion will be incomplete and stomach pain and constipation will result. *Pegen* cold energy may dominate due to an excess of cold food and drinks, leading to poor digestion. If there is too much *lung*, there is increased movement, and diarrhea may occur. However, if there is insufficient *lung*, the stomach is firm, and it is difficult to defecate. When *triba* is too strong, the stomach is soft and again, there is tendency towards diarrhea.

Tibetans classify **organs** as solid or hollow. The solid organs are the lungs, heart, liver, spleen, and kidneys. The hollow organs are the stomach, small intestines, large intestines, gall bladder, urinary bladder, and the *vesicles of the regenerative substances*, which refers to the genitals. What is important to understand here is that they are never considered to be entities that are functionally discrete.

It is important to understand that **the function creates the organ** and not the contrary. Therefore, if a body part is removed, *the function* nevertheless remains. This is why organ transplantation is possible. Moreover, the persistence of "phantom pain" described in Western medicine, for example, after amputation of an arm, can be explained by the continuing presence of the subtle energy in the invisible channels in the arm. This concept of function can also explain other phenomena, such as rewiring that occurs in the brain after injury, disease, or surgery.

Some parts of the body are more directly connected than others; for example, the eye is functionally linked to the liver, explaining the yellowing of eyes when the liver malfunctions, in the case of hepatitis and jaundice. Similarly, the heart is functionally connected to the tongue, and the kidneys to the ears.

It was not surprising to Tibetan doctors that relatively recently Western doctors began to understand the importance of good dental care and a healthy mouth in preventing some types of heart disease. Of course, the relationship between the eyes and the liver could not be ignored, because of the obvious connection between jaundice and the liver. On the other hand, in the West, it is not yet understood that the ear is functionally connected to the kidneys and in the case of ear discomfort, the kidneys may be the cause.

Jacques Haesaert explained: "This is also why I have often seen patients who were operated on, first for ear problems due to 'unknown causes', then operated on again, sometime later, for renal disorders. With knowledge of organic relationships, the Western physician would have understood that the origin of the ear disorder was not in the ears, but rather in the kidneys, and these operations could have been avoided. Moreover, the kidneys could have been treated before it became crucial to operate".

Tibetan medicine explains that a person is made up of *the five aggregates*, which are constantly changing, as they are *processes*. They are combined into a single working unit: a collection of physical and mental personal experiences, including feelings, ideas, thoughts, and habits. The five aggregates are form, sensation, perception, mental formation, and consciousness. An individual needs all of these five components in order to exist. They are defined as follows:

1. **Form** or matter corresponds to the physical body parts composed of the four basic elements.
2. **Sensation** or feeling is of three kinds—pleasant, unpleasant and indifferent. This is what we are experiencing when something happens to us.
3. **Perception** has the function of turning an indefinite experience into a definite, recognized, and identified experience. It is the mental process that registers and labels, for example, a color or shape of an object, or the emotion of fear.
4. **Mental formation** has a moral dimension. It is a conditioned response to the object we are experiencing.
5. **Consciousness** has the discrimination that physical elements are insufficient to produce experience. For example, the eye and the visible object alone cannot produce the *experience* of seeing. Consciousness is awareness of or sensitivity to an object.

In Buddhism, there is no difference between mind and consciousness. When asked to explain what the mind is, Lama Thubten Zopa Rinpoche responded: "What is the mind? It is a phenomenon that is not body, not substantial, has no form, no shape, no color, but, like a mirror, can clearly reflect objects."

For Western scientists, mind is something that emerges from brain activity in beings with sophisticated nervous systems. *Self* is then defined as the sum of all of one's memories and experiences.

Throughout our lives, we create the causes for our joy and distress. The foundation of Tibetan psychology is that all living beings, especially humans, are seeking perfect happiness and the elimination of suffering. Unfortunately, complete elimination of suffering is not possible—it is inherent in birth, aging, and death.

Tibetan doctors do all they can to relieve adversity. They follow a strict code of conduct that stresses sincere behavior and sympathy, which always accompanies the physical treatments. If a physician lacks compassion and awareness of patients' psychological needs, the consequences can be dire.

When my mother, who lived in the U.S.A., got to an advanced stage of diabetes with neuropathy and required kidney dialysis, she surely could not ignore that her condition was very serious and she was never going to get better, but was it really necessary for her primary doctor to answer her in the following way when she expressed her concern about increasing her pain medicine to include morphine? She told him that she was afraid of becoming addicted to it. He bluntly told her, with no preparation, "It's really not a problem, because you are terminal". These were his exact words.

We could call it lack of education, an absence of psychology, or simple lack of compassion. In any case, a lot of damage was done, which required much consolation to relieve her distress and profound sadness. Finally, what worked was to tell her, "Me too, I'm terminal. In fact, from the day we are born, we're all terminal! The way the doctor talked to you, makes me think he forgot this."

It was, nevertheless, a devastating experience, and it is my hope that all Western physicians are inspired by the compassion inherent in Tibetan medicine, so that no patient must ever hear, "There is nothing more I can do for you." There is always something, at least making the person as comfortable as possible and being attentive to their needs, with mindful listening and compassion.

Fear, and especially fear of death, are two important themes of psychology. Tibetan Buddhism teaches that by thinking about death every day, we can live fully significant lives. Instead of dreading death, we can accept it as an inevitable and normal occurrence and have compassion for ourselves. We can learn to pardon others and ourselves, perhaps feeling regret, but not guilt, which serves no purpose. Death is not a failure on the doctor's part, but is rather is a transition, an awakening from the dream of life and the road to rebirth.

In the West, death is not only something dreaded but is also something that many people are even unable to speak of. Tibetans realize that the moment of death can be positive, if a person can be prepared and die without regret and without fear. A person who is very old and/or very sick can ask themselves, "Now, is it better to stay, or to let go and pass away?" Likewise, as we accompany loved ones during their last days, we need to reflect on the fact that by imploring them to stay with us, we may be causing them suffering by holding them back.

The Tibetan physician is responsible for their patients during the last stage of life. They do not work to prolong life at any cost. They listen to their patients and help them remain serene in order to prepare themselves for death. It is very important that whoever accompanies the patient creates a warm and supportive environment, so that the patient can trust in their honesty in response to any questions they may pose.

CHAPTER 4

Conception, formation of the body, and childbirth

Tibetan medicine describes the whole process in detail, from conception to childbirth. The language used includes the non-Western terms of female and male *drops*, karma, reincarnation, the five elements, and the subtle energies. The subjects covered include; conditions for conception, factors that can prevent conception, signs of conception, abortion, determination of the sex of the baby, health of the pregnant woman, formation of the body, inherent and final signs of delivery, how to assure an easy birth, the birth process, and what to do after the birth.

Conception: a new life begins

Buddhists explain that physical events are not sufficient for a new being to develop. Specific causes and conditions need to be united, and when it no longer manifests it does not stop existing. It is not born and it does not die. It does not pass from the realm of being into the realm of non-being.

Conception is the moment when the consciousness enters into the "sperm-blood mixture" immediately following intercourse. The choice of the parents and the circumstances of time and place of conception are dependent on karma. Before entering into the "sperm-blood mixture", the being who has the karma to be born as a male feels aversion for his future father and desire for his future mother, and the being who has the karma to be born as a female feels aversion for the mother and desire for the father.

Freudian psychologists will smile at hearing this!

Highly evolved spiritual beings, including the Dalai Lama, can choose the moment of their reincarnation and their mother and father. They can also give indications, before their passing on, of where their birth will take place.

The subtle energy of desire is *lung* and the wish for life is what transports the consciousness, which is pushed by its accumulated karma, into the womb. The being "dies" in its actual state, which is either *bardo* or is an incarnation. *Bardo* is defined as an intermediate state between death and rebirth. The consciousness penetrates the sperm-ovum mixture and the energy of desire manifesting as *sokzin lung* enables this consciousness to associate with the five elements, which will be used to form its body using the *drops* of the mother and father, as intermediaries.

Jacques Haesaert explained that "the earth element forms the flesh, bones and olfactory organs and odors; water element forms blood, taste organs and the humidity and water of the body; fire element forms heat, clarity of complexion and sight organs. Air element forms the breath, touch, and physical perceptions such as hot and cold. Space element forms the body's cavities, hearing organs and sounds. The consciousness's sokzin lung is associated with the space element." The consciousness does not reside in a particular site in the body, but it is represented in the heart.

In Figure 7, we find all these elements needed for the coming into existence of a new being. We also find the clear light mind, which is the subtlest level of mind. It is the nature of mind experienced in deep sleep and death. It has the qualities that we would call Buddha-nature and thanks to this, everyone can become a Buddha, an enlightened being free from ignorance.

Even if one does not believe in reincarnation, it is interesting to understand the Tibetan explanation.

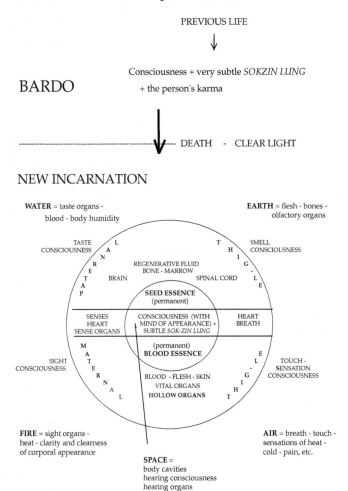

Figure 7. Reincarnation and formation of the body under the control of the five *lung* energies.

Conditions for conception

The male and female components, of good quality, and favorable conditions must be united in order for fertilization to occur. Defective sperm, a defective *egg* (the regenerative fluid plus *blood* energy), a defective womb, inappropriate karma, a defect in one or more of the five elements, or unfavorable astrological influences can all prevent conception.

Healthy sperm is white, heavy, sweet, and abundant. The subtle energy responsible for poor quality sperm can be determined and treatment can be given.

There are three categories of defects of the *egg*. In the first category of maternal disorders, the blood is dark and has a solid appearance. The mother feels pain in the lower parts of the body, the waist, and breasts and may have irregular menstruation. In cases of the second category, menstrual blood is yellowish and foul-smelling. The woman may have some fever and headache. Disorders of the third category are characterized by thin, odorless menstrual blood. There are often whitish discharges during or after menstruation, and a feeling of fatigue and agitation.

A defective womb may also be responsible for sterility. A physical deformation of the uterus may prevent the egg from remaining implanted. Medicines are applied directly onto the woman's body. If the cause is an excess of cold, her body should always be kept sufficiently warm. An ointment containing nutmeg is applied to the whole region of the abdomen. and internal medicine is given. In the case of hot disorders, a refreshing medicine is given.

In general, a woman who is trying to conceive a child needs to keep the region of her abdomen and lower back warm, even in the summer. It is better to not take baths or showers every day in order to avoid excessive physical contact with water and cold temperatures. Women may wash themselves with a washcloth daily and shower less often. They are advised to avoid all alcoholic drinks and take care to get appropriate nutrients. Warm, cooked foods and hot drinks are recommended.

I highly recommend Dr. Lobsang Shrestha 's very informative and practical book, *Healthy Child and Mother, Happy Family* (*see* Suggested reading) as well as the book of teachings by Jacques Haesaert.

Determination of the baby's sex

The information provided by Tibetan medicine is precise and detailed, and it may sound unusual to our Western ears. Moreover, the reader will probably be surprised by the information about which days a girl or boy child is likely to be conceived and how to determine the sex of the child, very early in the pregnancy.

The texts describe the moments in the woman's menstrual cycle when a child can be conceived, as well as the specific moments to conceive a male or female child. The texts state that if sexual relations occur the first three days of the period or on the 11th of the twelve days following the period, a boy cannot be conceived. If the relations take place the 1st, 3rd, 7th or 9th day of this twelve-day period, a boy will be conceived. When relations occur on the 2nd, 4th, 6th, 8th, 10th and 12th day, a girl will be conceived.

There are other methods that can be employed if, specifically, a boy or girl is desired. A physician can even determine the probable sex of a baby during pregnancy. A physician can also determine the probable sex of a baby before conception, by taking the parents' pulses. The methods for, and information provided by, reading pulses are very complex, as explained in Chapter 10—Symptoms and Diagnosis.

Formation of the body

Each stage of development of the baby is described in detail in the texts. First, *sok lung* energy and the future baby's consciousness connect to the elements to begin to form its body. Other subtle energies are then made to direct the formation of each new function, organ, and other parts of the body.

After conception, the umbilical cord emerges from the nucleus of the embryo, which then develops into a fetus that grows and develops for thirty-eight weeks.

During the first week, the consistency of the embryo is like curdled milk and in the second week, the embryonic mixture thickens. The embryo is really formed at this moment. During the third week it hardens even more into the consistency of yogurt.

The events of the following weeks are all described up to the 38th week, at which point the child turns over in its mother's womb and moves down, in preparation for birth.

Health of the pregnant woman and the birth process

It cannot be stressed enough that it is vital to take very good care of the mother, so the pregnancy can proceed under optimal conditions. Dr. Lobsang Shrestha explains that she should receive special care and stay free from any negativity, including immoral people. Excesses should be avoided and specific food should be given to help regain her strength after childbirth. Particular attention is also given to the child, to avoid problems later in life.

The role of high-quality food for the mother is emphasized. Teachings go so far as to say that during gestation, the mother should avoid eating food given to her by people of questionable morality. Specific spiritual practices and blessings from lamas are also undertaken in Tibet. Nourishing, healthy food should be eaten in moderate amounts. The mother should avoid alcohol; sour, heavy, and spicy foods that have a burning taste; all food or medicine that cause constipation, purgation, or vomiting; vaginal douching; and treatments that cause loss of blood, such as surgery, as they may kill the fetus.

Pregnant women are cautioned to avoid hard work and encouraged to sleep. They should nevertheless remain active, performing light tasks and moderate exercise, such as walking, for good blood circulation.

Sexual relations are permitted during the first eight months of pregnancy; however, great caution must be taken and movements must be very gentle during the seventh and eighth months. Relations are forbidden during the ninth month because they may affect the energy of the developing infant, creating damage to the brain.

When the moment of birth is near, the mother is given very nourishing food, such as bone marrow soup, milk, rice and butter. She should avoid onions and garlic that affect muscle relaxation because of their burning and acidic properties. It is said that these nutrients also cause laziness of the child in the womb, weakening its power to help in the birth process and delaying the contractions.

There are methods, including spiritual practices, that can provide relief, in the case of a long and difficult birth, and other practices are done immediately after birth in Tibet. After childbirth, the new mother should refrain from taking showers; humidity and cold can cause health problems that manifest later in life.

CHAPTER 5

What is health?

Health is defined by more than being free from illness or injury. It is a state of physical, mental, emotional, spiritual, and social well-being and equilibrium. Tibetan medicine explains that the key is to keep the three subtle energies balanced. Health is also defined by the presence of the correct amount of warm energy in the body, rather than just the absence of pain or wounds, infection, or degeneration.

Living in harmony with all beings and with nature, abstaining from harmful behavior, inappropriate foods and negative emotions, and feeling satisfied with our lives help to maintain this equilibrium.

This balance of the three energies is affected by many factors, including age, lifestyle, emotions, and behavior, which includes our actions, words, and thoughts. Moreover, the seasons, climate, and other environmental factors also influence health. Good physician-patient relations and confidence in the treatments are also important for health and healing.

Buddhists explain that another factor in health and disease is karma. When we are experiencing good health, one of the factors is thus the accumulation of positive actions from earlier in our lives or past lives. Nevertheless, many bad things happen to "good" people. People fall ill for many reasons. We all know of such cases and feel a sense of injustice that such a kind person faces overwhelming difficulties that they did not deserve. Karma can be the explanation.

Once a malady or any other unfortunate event occurs, the negative karma that was responsible for it is used up and finished. However, this does not mean that the patient should not be treated!

Events we perceive as negative can nevertheless have positive aspects. Sometimes our bodies help us remain healthy by manifesting great fatigue to get us to stay home and relax, so sickness does not result from over-work and stress. A small accident or undesired event may prevent a more serious one from occurring. A moment of inattention that results in a car accident, without consequences, can be a wake-up call to drive more carefully.

If we can identify the positive aspect of an event, the negative side is much easier to bear. Many cancer patients have told me, in the course of my hospice visits, that something very strong came out of their disease that changed their lives in a very positive way, notably, understanding what is really important in life. They realized that they had been wasting a lot of their time and energy of this precious life on frivolities rather than the essential, including spending more time with loved ones.

I quote the Dalai Lama: "Every day, think as you wake up, today I am fortunate to be alive, I have a precious human life, I am not going to waste it. I am going to use all my energies to develop myself, to expand my heart out to others and achieve enlightenment for the benefit of all beings. I am going to have kind thoughts towards others, I am not going to get angry or think badly about others. I am going to benefit others as much as I can."

CHAPTER 6

Behavior and nutrition

The information concerning these important topics may prove the most useful for the reader who is a novice to Tibetan medicine. Lifestyle factors and nutrition play incredibly important roles in maintaining health. Most health problems can be either directly or indirectly traced to poor nutrition or lifestyle choices. The first form of treatment in Tibetan medicine is thus changing what a patient eats and/or does. If this is not sufficient, then the use of medicines is considered.

Having a good attitude and adapting our activities and behavior to the climate, our age, and our present situation help keep us well. An awareness and mindfulness of each moment of our lives is important, whether we are eating, walking, lying down, doing sport, or working. Getting sufficient sleep is essential. Allowing for time to relax and meditate is also important.

An example of behavior that can bring harmony and peace, instead of leading a couple to divorce, is considering what we thought to be a default in one's mate as a quality, instead! This includes not always trying to change our partners to meet our criteria, but rather accept them as they are. It is also a big step in the right direction to understand that no one except ourselves can be responsible for our own happiness.

Appropriate behavior according to the season

We are better off adjusting to seasonal changes, as animals and plants do, throughout the year. Wearing appropriate clothing and changing ambient temperatures are not sufficient. It is clear that some behavior, such as walking, is very good in all seasons, but different times of the year are better for more or less vigorous activities.

According to the season and specific periods of each season, each subtle energy either *accumulates*, *manifests*, or *is pacified*, as illustrated by Jacques Haesaert in Figure 8: The seasonal cycle of the energies. We are, therefore, more prone to come down with a certain disorder during a specific time of the year. Even doses of some Western medicines, such as those for the thyroid, often need adjusting.

Timing is one of the important factors in disease. This includes the age of the person, the season, and time of day, all of which determine what is appropriate behavior. *Lung* disorders arise especially in summer, in the evening and just before dawn. *Triba* disorders arise especially in autumn, in the afternoon and at night. *Pegen* disorders arise especially in spring, at twilight and dawn. This means that it is good to adapt our nutrition and behavior. Healthy food for a sedentary elderly person living in the mountains in winter is very different from that needed by an adolescent living by the sea in summer.

Altitude, climate, and weather all affect the three energies in different ways. There are three weather conditions: heat, cold, and precipitation. If they are over-abundant in any given season, they are called excessive; if they lack, they are insufficient. If it is cold in the warm season or vice versa, or if it rains in the dry season, these conditions are called perverse. Harsh weather conditions and wind contribute to *lung* disorders. Cold is a factor in their sudden appearance and heat pacifies them. Heat is a cause of *triba* perturbance, while conditions such as heaviness combined with cold provoke *pegen* disturbances.

Since *pegen*, the energy of water and earth, increases in spring, it is best to avoid extensive contact with water. For most people, a daily shower is not recommended. However, avoiding access to water does not apply to the young, who need more *pegen*. In spring, it is beneficial to exercise more. It is also the ideal time to begin practicing yoga.

Swimming is good in summer to calm *triba*, the energy of fire. Meditating is always beneficial, but more is recommended in summer. It is not the good season for saunas because they are so hot. Warming food and drink such as alcohol, inappropriate conduct, violent or perturbing actions or staying for long periods in the sun all contribute to hot disorders. Symptoms include a bitter taste in the mouth, headache, and excessive body heat. These symptoms are stronger during digestion. A cool environment and refreshing food can relieve these symptoms. However, it is not advised to stay in air-conditioned spaces or drink ice cold beverages, even in the summer, because of the cooling effect on the *digestive fire*, which creates stomach problems.

Certain seasons are better for having more sex than others, and the best time is after the autumn equinox. Sex is especially good for people with dominant *lung*, the energy of wind and movement. It is very good to swim in the fall. Fasting should not be undertaken unless the doctor prescribes it; but if it is recommended, the best season for it is autumn. Likewise, this is the best season for thermal cures.

Winter is not a good time to do rigorous sports or activities. However, persons who have a strong constitution and those who eat rich and oily foods should stay relatively active in winter. Think of the animals that hibernate in winter. We too would be better off slowing down.

Our bodies adjust to the external cold and block the body pores to keep the heat inside the body. This increase in the inner heat enhances the power of the "digestive fire", which means that food is digested faster. In order for the body to remain at an optimal temperature for digestion and not endanger the body, appropriate diet and behavior should be maintained in healthy balance.

Wearing light clothes in winter is a contributing factor to disease, as it results in an increase in *lung* and a decrease in *triba*. This kind of behavior is particularly harmful to women who hope to become pregnant. It is important for them to keep the whole area of the abdomen and lower back warm, especially in this season.

The later part of winter is usually colder and more humid than early winter. *Pegen* energy accumulates in the body and then manifests in the spring, as the body and the earth begin to warm up. In later spring and summer, the earth and body warm up, and heat deeply penetrates the body. In autumn, the heat of the sun and external heat gradually decrease, but the internal heat remains strong.

Variation of temperatures is a natural method of maintaining balance of the three energies and normal bodily functions. The seasons thus give the power of movement to circulate the energy flow throughout the body, keeping the organs and tissues healthy. When the body is unhealthy, blockages and symptoms appear and then eventually the disease is expulsed.

These seasonal rhythms are vital for us, and by observing nature, we can better understand the importance of making changes. There is a cycle created during the year in the human body by movement of the three subtle energies, parallel to the cycle that occurs in plants.

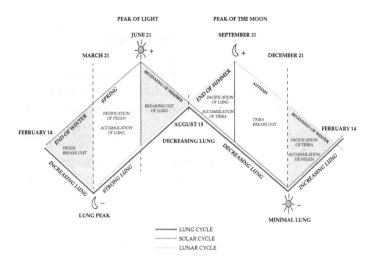

Figure 8. The seasonal cycle of the energies.

In fact, the body can be compared to a tree, *The Tree of Life*, and its growth is similar to ours. We find analogies between the body and the tree of life as follows:

- Roots of the tree represent bones and flesh and provide structure.
- Leaves represent hair on the head, body hair, and nails.
- The fruits are the five vital organs.
- The *heart* represents bone marrow.
- The resin and sap represent the circulatory and nervous systems.
- Branches represent limbs.
- The bark represents skin.

In Figure 9, we see which elements dominate during the four seasons, the correlation between body components and parts of the tree, and examples of substances used as treatments.

This comparison between the body and *The Tree of Life*, important in Tibetan medicine, confirms the notion of "like heals like" as explained in homeopathy, as well as by the Swiss physician, Paracelsus in the 1500s. He wrote that nature marks each growth according to its curative benefit and that plants resembling various parts of the body can be used to treat ailments of those body parts. Similarly, the Doctrine of Signatures, dating from the time of early Greek physicians, states that herbs resembling various parts of the body can be used to treat diseases of those body parts. There are many examples of this in nature. To cite

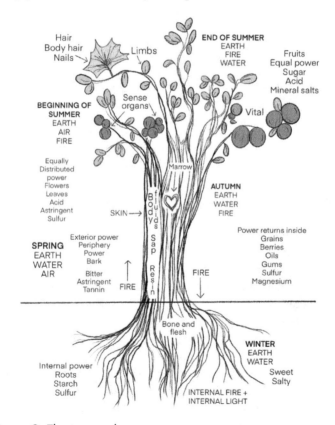

Figure 9. The tree and man.

one example, Poulose and colleagues (2014) showed that polyphenolic compounds found in walnuts reduce the oxidant and inflammatory load on brain cells and also improve signaling between neurons, increase neurogenesis, and enhance sequestration of insoluble toxic protein aggregates.

Beneficial medical substances can also be found in minerals, because *everything* in the universe is interrelated.

How behavior leads to disease

Insufficient sleep, remaining for a long time in a windy place, travelling by plane, and experiencing great suffering and strong emotions are conditions contributing to *lung* disorders, characterized by lightness and movement. Other conditions include forcing muscles to contract or relax while urinating, defecating, coughing or sneezing. Holding your breath or retaining abdominal gas can also be harmful.

It is recommended that a person with a *lung* disorder stay sufficiently covered, in a warm place, in the company of pleasant companions. One should not exert oneself excessively on an empty stomach. Tai Chi Chuan is particularly beneficial to anchor the person to the ground in order to counter the lightness and wind of *lung*.

It is better for a patient suffering from a *triba* disorder, associated with excess heat, to stay in cool places and not partake in vigorous or violent activities. Staying calm and avoiding difficult persons and circumstances which are annoying are helpful.

Inactivity and lying for long periods on humid grass contribute to *pegen* disorders, which are associated with fluids, heaviness, and the cold. Someone with such a disorder may experience digestive difficulties. It is better for them to stay in a warm place and take a walk after eating. Remaining physically active is especially important in winter and spring.

Our pores open in a sauna and a lot of cold energy can enter the body, after stepping out. Therefore, it is good to massage the body with warm oil after the sauna.

General behavior to avoid

Disease is more prevalent in dirty places, so one should keep one's house clean, with frequent aeration. Polluted places should be avoided when possible and especially during physical activity. The risks of jogging in a polluted city can be greater than its benefits.

Air conditioning and direct ventilation from a fan should be avoided. As mentioned before, not getting enough sleep is very harmful and sleeping eight hours per night is recommended. Over-stimulating activities, such as playing violent video games or watching television programs, are not conducive to good sleep. Overheating the bedroom makes sleep more difficult. Vaporising essential oils, such as lavender, has a calming effect. It is also helpful to meditate before going to bed.

Appropriate behavior and limiting food intake later than early evening could greatly reduce the need for sleeping pills, which are grossly over-prescribed in France, and throughout the Western world.

A good breakfast and a well-nourishing meal are recommended at lunchtime. This is the time to eat high protein foods. It is better to eat a light dinner, early in the evening.

Dr. Lobsang Shrestha explains that menstruating women who expose themselves to a lot of humidity by showering and bathing causes health problems later in life, including menopause. Women also create conditions for disorders by not removing their bras while sleeping, due to the pressure applied to the region of the breasts, especially if there is wire in the bra, which increases the compression.

The importance of caring for babies properly cannot be stressed enough. It can be very dangerous to move a baby roughly, shake it, or lift it into the air. Serious irreversible consequences may be induced. Their fragile organs can move out of position putting the life of the child in danger.

Foods adapted to the individual's needs

Tibetan medicine treats each person as a unique case. Nonetheless, there are guidelines that lead to greater well-being and vitality, including eating nutritionally-balanced, natural foods and drinks and eating at the correct times.

The typical American diet, rich in prepared, processed food and ice cold, sweetened bottled drinks and large quantities of coffee, is the antithesis of what Tibetan medicine advises. Most foods consumed are full of additives as well as high salt concentrations and added sugar, or harmful substitutes such as aspartame. Prepared foods on the shelves of food shops contain high fructose corn syrup, added in order to increase the "desirability" of the product, but which is rapidly converted to fat and stored. Its consumption mirrors the increase in obesity across the USA and some other countries. Moreover, high fructose corn syrup, unlike other foods, does not lead to a rise in leptin, a hormone that helps us feel full. It is important to read the list of ingredients before buying food; it can help the buyer make better, informed choices and remove the attraction of unhealthy foods.

A large part of many food budgets are spent on restaurant and take-out food, although most restaurants use poor quality ingredients, likely to contain pesticides and other harmful chemicals to save money. Moreover, many people eat mostly prepared, stored, refrigerated and frozen food, which has lost most of its essence and is, therefore, less capable of satisfying hunger. Although many Westerners prefer milk that is fat-free, thinking that the milk fat is adding useless calories to their diet, this milk is difficult to digest and warmed whole milk is much healthier. Likewise, most customers choose yogurt with high sugar and fruit content, finding it more prevalent on shelves in food stores than plain yogurt, and thinking that it is good for health.

The main problem is the accessibility of the unhealthy foods and the fact that they appear to be the *normal* things to eat, because everyone else is doing the same thing and because of misleading publicity. Rarely do we take into account the long-term effects of our food choices, thinking instead of only what we like and what tastes delicious.

There are always good alternatives. For example, unhealthy salad dressings can be easily substituted with virgin olive oil with or without a bit of lemon. An easy way to avoid over-salting food is to use a commercial mixture of salt that contains potassium and magnesium chloride, instead of just sodium chloride, or to use herbal substitutes. Moreover, one gets the benefit of the other ingredients. Honey, in moderate amounts, or stevia (a sweetener derived from the leaves of the plant species *Stevia rebaudiana*) can be used in the place of sugar.

The right choice of food and drink is part of preventive medicine and is important for healing processes. Cold and hot qualities, taste, smell, and other qualities of foods determine their effects on the three subtle energies. A Tibetan doctor always advises his patients on nutrition according to which of the three energies are affected, and according to whether the affliction is hot or cold in nature.

In the same way as for behavior, it is advised to make food choices based on our present state, age, place of residence, usual activities, season, climate, weather, and the time of day. Total food intake needs to be reduced as we age, for all metabolic processes slow down. If we continue to eat as much as when we were young, most of us will most likely gain weight and belly fat. Fresh organic milk is an excellent food for babies and children, while not particularly recommended for adults, although in many cases it is not contra-indicated if one likes it and it is not drunk cold. However, the elderly and persons with low energy levels benefit greatly from easily digestible fresh, boiled, organic whole milk. Our tastes change with age and it is good to listen to our cravings because they can sometimes tell us what we need at that moment.

Tibetan doctors are not fans of soy milk, which has no particular advantage and lacks the good qualities of milk. Eating local, in-season, fresh organic food whenever possible is always best. Nature provides us with what we need during each season.

It is better to avoid raw food, including salads, in winter. In general, warm cooked foods are better than raw and cold foods, which should at least be accompanied by some that are warm. This is true for many reasons.

- The cold perturbs the *digestive fire* resulting in stomach disorders.
- Heat destroys harmful micro-organisms.
- Heat also inactivates some toxins.
- Cooking also softens and renders the food more digestible, particularly onions and sweet peppers.

Of course, avoiding dogma, refreshing food can be advised in cases of excess *triba* energy.

Refrigerated food acquires, over time, the cold and heavy *pegen* qualities. This energy is also associated with darkness, immobility, and water, whereas food left in the open air and light, even if it is cold, acquires the quality of lightness, as opposed to heaviness. Potatoes, however, should be always stored in the dark, to avoid sprouting and turning green, which creates toxic products.

Meat and fish consumption is not usually advised because of the suffering to which the animals are subjected—See the excellent book by Matthieu Richard, *A Plea for the Animals: The Moral Philosophy and Evolutionary Imperative to Treat All Beings with Compassion*. However, once again, dogma and judgment should be avoided. After childbirth or after certain serious medical disorders, specific animal products can be recommended. Meat has therapeutic properties that differ according to the species, but also according to the climate where the animal lives and what it eats. In general, it is advised to avoid non-organic chicken and any kind of pork.

Dr. Lobsang Shrestha teaches that the most nutritive food, bone-marrow broth, is particularly recommended in the case of extreme weakness and after childbirth. It is prepared by boiling large bovine bones and filtering the broth, which can be consumed with added rice or pasta, vegetables, nuts, sesame seeds, and spices, such as cardamom, nutmeg, and cumin. It is the most nutritive food.

It is important that vegetarians and vegans take special care to include beans, lentils, chickpeas, seeds, all kinds of nuts, and oils in their diets. For a vegetarian, fresh whole milk and butter are also recommended. Mushrooms are a very good substitute for meat. With proper choices, there are no disadvantages to these diets for most people.

Addiction to substances such as alcohol and caffeine can create a lot of problems. Instead of thinking about long-term effects, we think of the short-term pleasure. If it is too difficult to abstain from consuming them, we can at least limit them. Coffee with milk is less harmful.

Drinking ice cold beverages is not only very bad for digestion; they do not even satisfy one's thirst as well as warm ones, even in the heat of the summer. Indians have always known and applied this wisdom, choosing warm chai, a flavored tea beverage, instead.

A particularly harmful habit is to drink a glass of bottled orange juice every day, straight from the refrigerator as part of breakfast, because it is sour and cold. It is even worse when combined with a bowl of cereal with cold milk. It is much better to drink room temperature, freshly pressed juice from ripe fruit, between meals.

It is not necessary to be a scholar in Tibetan medicine to understand that drinking anything sweetened and full of caffeine is unhealthy. The enormous consumption of drinks with a lot of sugar, including sodas, lemonades, bottled iced tea, and energy drinks, partly explains the obesity epidemic. Good sense would dictate drinking warm water instead. This also eliminates the intake of sugar substitutes that have undesirable effects, except for natural products like honey and stevia. Even the food budget benefits from making water one's preferred beverage! A cup of hot water first thing in the morning is best. It hydrates and warms the body, reducing the "need" for coffee. A lot of the effects that a person thinks are coming from morning coffee or tea come, in fact, from the temperature of the water. During sleep, the body cools down and warming it up in the morning makes us feel more awake. This warm water in the morning is especially good for a pregnant woman or a woman who hopes to conceive and wants to cut down or eliminate her consumption of coffee. It is even recommended to continue drinking warm water throughout the day and during meals.

As described earlier, it is best to eat nutritious meals early in the day, and eat lightly in the evening, as early as possible. A warm breakfast and a very nourishing lunch are recommended. Midday is the best time to eat rich and heavy foods because we are most active during the day, and our metabolism peaks. Lunch consisting mostly of a salad or a small cold sandwich is not sufficient, even in summer. At night, our metabolism is slowed down, so digestion takes longer. This is why eating big meals late in the evening contributes to weight gain. This knowledge is not restricted to Tibetan medicine; more and more studies are being done on this subject. A light, early dinner can include a soup, a small portion of rice or pasta in small quantities, or vegetables. Fruit is best eaten between meals.

What and how we eat, how much, as well as the conditions in which we eat all affect our health. Overeating causes problems because it limits movement of the nutrients in the digestive tract. Ideally, our food and drink should be 2/3 solid and 1/3 liquid. The stomach should ideally be 3/4 full + 1/4 empty, after a meal. This is optimal for digestion because it enables the passage of the food components during their transformation in the digestive system.

Food is also assimilated better when we eat mindfully, with enjoyment, without distractive thoughts and activities. Therefore, when eating, it is recommended to just eat and not do something else at the same time. Eating in a calm, pleasant atmosphere enables the person to fully benefit from the food. It is good to eat slowly and remember to give thanks to whoever provided the food as well as to the animals whose sacrifice was their very own lives. A moment of rest is good after meals, instead of rapidly resuming activities or taking a cold bath.

Eating at regular intervals is important. Tibetans use the analogy of cooking food in a pot on the stove. If nothing is put into an empty stomach (the pot), the digestive energy can become destructive, especially in winter, when digestive fire is particularly powerful. Likewise, if food enters the stomach when there is not enough hot energy because of too little *triba*, digestion will be difficult (the food in the pot will not cook). In both cases, repetitive errors lead to serious or chronic disorders.

One cannot emphasize enough the indispensable development of the faculty of intuition. It is even said that all the difference between a physician of great intelligence and one of average or mediocre intelligence is his faculty of intuition. Likewise, developing our intuition can bring us great benefit. In fact, intelligence does not signify intellect but rather global comprehension, which is the fruit of intuitive intelligence.

If we "listen" to our bodies, and try to understand our cravings, we can get information about what our choice of food should be. This is not about a need that we have created, for example, for a glass of wine right after work. Good sense tells us if we often have stomach discomfort with a feeling of too much acidity, it is time to greatly reduce coffee and sour foods, such as unripe fruit and choose instead some unctuous and inherently sweet food (not sugared food). In cold weather, we are tempted by a warm soup, rather than a salad. A Tibetan doctor may use the example of a person with a *lung* disturbance developing a desire for the smooth quality of butter as one of the aggravating qualities of *lung* is coarseness, the opposite.

The notion of *du-chi* is also important in Tibetan medicine. *Du-chi* means "nectar-poison". This means that any substance, including any nutrient, has the potential of *du* and *chi* and circumstance is what determines which of the two it is. Eating great excesses of spinach or eating many Brazil nuts becomes dangerous, because spinach contains a substantial amount of oxalic acid, and Brazil nuts a have high selenium content. Very small amounts of processed mercury, wisely used, can be therapeutic, in specific cases. This is telling us that we should exercise moderation, the Buddhist notion of the "middle road": not too much and not too little, avoiding excesses in everything we do.

Foods for the three dominant energy types

It is recommended that each person eat the foods appropriate for their dominant energy type as well as their present energetic state. For example, a person with the heat of dominant *triba* is advised to limit very warming food—such as certain spices—and choose instead coriander and other seasonings with cooling qualities. The effects of a food on the three subtle energies also depend upon the proportion of the five elements that it contains.

Specific conditions leading to the appearance of hot disorders include excessive food or medicine that is spicy hot, salty, or oily. Similarly, if a person is enduring a period of excessive anger and hatred, or carrying out hard physical work during warm weather, *triba* can increase to excess. Accordingly, sweet, astringent, and refreshing foods such as raw freshly-prepared juices or tofu are recommended. Foods to avoid or limit include meat, garlic, butter, or brown sugar, as well as all alcohol. This may sound strange because one is taught that the more active one is, the more consistent food should be. However, here we are talking about qualities of food and not just calories.

Remedies for a person with a *triba* disorder have sweet, bitter, and refreshing qualities. Recommended foods include yogurt, milk, fresh butter, barley, spinach, and dandelion—used here as a vegetable though sometimes used as medicine.

Warm and cooked food, instead of raw and cold food, is good for a person with a light, *lung* constitution or a temporary excess of *lung*. The specific conditions causing the appearance of *lung* disorders include an excess of foods or medicines that are light, bitter, or coarse. A person with this dominant energy is advised to avoid unripe fruits, black coffee, soy sauce, vinegar, and all food preserved in vinegar, such as pickles. Raw and cold foods are harmful for persons with dominant *lung* or temporary *lung* excess, and missing meals worsens their condition. Symptoms are most evident when the patient is hungry, so nourishing and oily food is beneficial for persons with symptoms of excess *lung*. Sweet and salty foods are recommended. Suitable foods include honey, avocados, meat, vegetables, sesame oil, and butter. Other recommended substances include certain meats, garlic, onions, and warm whole milk.

The consumption of oily and heavy food, as well as overeating, or eating and then starting again to eat before digestion is completed are specific conditions that result in the appearance of disorders of *pegen*, the heavy, slow, and cold energy. This is also true for eating burned food, cold leftovers, and all cold beverages such as low-fat milk. Persons with this dominant energy are advised to consume warming foods that are easy to digest. Food with inherent qualities of acrid, rough, and light are recommended. Reasonable quantities of curry, chili peppers, and rice are particularly good.

Some foods are particularly useful to help balance the three energies. These include carrots and cheese in moderation. It is beyond the scope of this book to give detailed food lists. Examples of foods to be recommended or avoided in the case of energy imbalances are given below. In the case of excess of two subtle energies, some of these foods are excluded and others favored.

EXAMPLES OF RECOMMANDED FOODS IN THE CASE OF ENERGY IMBALANCE

Lung
Good for calming the light *lung* energy of movement
- Tastes: sweet, salty
- Warming, moistening qualities; protein, carbohydrates
- Examples: grains, cereals, beans, brown rice, cooked onions and garlic, animal products, such as butter and cheese, bone marrow soup, mushrooms, warm milk, hot peppers, cooked vegetables, ginger, cardamom, nutmeg, clove, hot tea

Bad for *lung* symptoms
- Cold food, raw food, frozen foods
- Food with cold quality e.g. cucumber, zucchini, lettuce, cabbage
- Acidic food like unripe fruit, vinegar, young wine, soft drinks, coffee, soy sauce

Triba
Good for calming the hot *triba* energy
- Tastes: bitter, sweet, astringent
- Cooling quality
- Fruits, especially lemon and papaya, most vegetables, green beans, cereals, grains, yogurt, rice, light herbal tea, beans

Bad for *triba* symptoms
- Beef, hot curry, blue cheese, fermented food, vinegar, eggs garlic, soft drinks, alcohol, coffee, some nuts, chili

Pegen
Good for calming the cold, heavy *pegen* energy
- Tastes: pungent, bitter, astringent
- Warming, drying qualities
- Light, easy to digest food, cooked vegetables, bone marrow soup, hot peppers, pomegranate, mango, banana, eggs, spices such as ginger, cardamom, nutmeg, cumin, garlic

Bad for *pegen* symptoms
- Raw, heavy, cold food, beer, sugar, soft drinks, coffee, green pepper, cucumbers, zucchini, lettuce, fermented food

Qualities and classification of food

It is very important to understand how food choices affect our health. In general, it can be said that Westerners would be better off consuming less cold and acidic foods, which in the long-term are causative of chronic disease development.

Each type of food is inherently made up of a certain proportion of the five elements, and is of a "cold" or "hot" nature. The term "cold food" refers as much to the power of the food as to its temperature. We can eat food that is hot in temperature but has cold power. As one would expect, the same food at a cold temperature has even more cold power. A cucumber is a good example of a food that is cold in quality.

Other qualities include fresh, light, heavy, unctuous, acidifying, rough, and fluid. Qualities of food depend on several criteria; smell, where and when the food grows or the animal is raised, and when and how the food is harvested and stored. Foods have qualities that depend on how the food is prepared. For example, boiled eggs have a cooling effect and aid in treating hot disorders, while fried eggs are warming and worsen them. The species of the animal laying an egg also confers specific qualities to it. Similarly, milk from different species has very different qualities.

The most important quality of food is taste. The sweet, sour, salty, bitter, pungent, and astringent tastes affect the three subtle energies. Texture and the proportion of the five elements are also characteristics that determine the effects of a food. For example, food with high water and earth content increase *pegen*, the energy of liquids including mucus; therefore, foods that increase this subtle energy aggravate the discomfort of having too much mucus, for example, when we have a cold or sinus problem.

People with discomfort due to excessive stomach acidity are advised to avoid anything with vinegar, including certain salad dressings, pickles, and sauerkraut. Soy sauce and young wines are also acidic. To reduce the acidity of tomatoes, the peel can be discarded. Like all fruits, they should be ripe.

Foods are divided into five groups: grains, oils, meats, vegetables, and liquids.

Grains of leguminous plants, such as beans and lentils are not described in the medical texts but are included in oral teachings of Tibetan and Ayurvedic medicine. They are excellent sources of protein and other nutrients, but can create flatulence. Eaten in large quantities or fried, they can cause constipation. It is, therefore, advised to eat them well cooked, with ingredients that counter these effects, as explained below.

Peas have a sweet taste and are astringent and slightly bitter. They have cooling and light qualities. Chickpeas cause less flatulence than other peas. When they are sprouted, they are easier to assimilate and are then beneficial for the three energies. Soy beans have both sweet and bitter tastes. Beans are sweet, astringent. Black lentils have a sweet taste. Their consummation is especially recommended in winter when they are cooked with other ingredients beneficial for the light, wind energy of *lung*. Orange lentils have some different effects since they have astringent and sweet tastes.

It is especially important for vegetarians and vegans to eat beans, lentils and chickpeas, rich in proteins. The unwanted side effects are controlled by having a balanced diet. They should be sufficiently cooked and not be eaten every day. It is best to always cook them with ingredients that limit the formation of gas, such as cumin, lemon juice, oil, butter, onions, and garlic.

Cereals such as wheat, rice, and barley have sweet, cooling, and softening effects. They are especially good for *lung* disorders. Rice is light and easy to digest. It is recommended for diarrhea and nausea. Millet, wheat, and barley are heavy. Overweight persons are advised to stop eating white bread and refined cereals, in general.

Oils have a sweet taste and heavy and refreshing qualities. Animal fats are more warming than oils extracted from most plants. Oils are especially important for young children, the elderly, anyone who is weak or convalescing, and anyone who has lost a lot of blood, such as women with heavy menstruation.

Butter is an important oil, and its effects greatly vary according to its origin and age. As butter ages, it becomes more warming, while fresh butter is more cooling. Excessively old butter should not be eaten.

Westerners can profit from the availability of virgin, cold-pressed olive oil, sesame, walnut, and flax seed oils, as well as fish and other oils. The production of palm oil has a very negative impact on the environment, and this oil is unfortunately present in many prepared food products. Butter, rich in vitamin E and other nutrients, should not be systematically substituted with margarine. Recent scientific publications have concluded that previous advice to strictly limit the intake of butter due to high levels of cholesterol does not apply to everyone. In a study conducted by Engel and Tholstrup (2015), they concluded that "hypercholesterolemic people should keep their consumption of butter to a minimum, whereas moderate butter intake may be considered part of the diet in the normo-cholesterolemic population." Moreover, we must be aware of what works for the patient. For example, fresh butter is sometimes recommended for *triba* disorders.

The qualities of meat depend not only on the species but also on what the animals eat, where they are raised, their age, how the meat is prepared, and the part of the animal it comes from. The meat of animals living at low altitudes is hot in quality and heavy and oily, while the meat of animals living at intermediate altitudes is lighter. That of wild animals is light, rough, and warming. The method of cooking greatly influences its effects. In general, cooking makes meat lighter and easier to digest. However, fried meat is heavy and harder to digest.

Most vegetables are warm and light when they grow in a dry region and cold when they grow in a humid region; however, altitude and temperature also play a role. At high altitudes, vegetables are usually cooling and light. They are generally more warming and heavier when grown on lowlands. The ripeness and freshness of vegetables greatly affect their qualities. Fresh vegetables, as opposed to frozen, are recommended.

Green vegetables help to clean the intestines and the urinary tract and are beneficial in the case of fever. However, an excess in the spring season causes *lung* energy to stagnate, provoking swelling of the stomach. These undesirable effects can be avoided by cooking green vegetables; they become lighter, warmer, and more tender. Therefore, raw vegetables should always be eaten in moderate quantities and balanced with cooked vegetables and food such as butter or oil to counterbalance the effects on *lung*.

There are so many types of vegetables that it is only possible to describe some of them here. Moreover, their properties vary, depending on how they are prepared and with which other foods they are eaten. For example, cabbage, cauliflower, aubergine, and radishes can adsorb a lot of fat. Adding the heavy qualities of fats to warming qualities of some foods, such as aubergine, can increase hot disorders, but can be very useful in the case of an excess of the light energy *lung*.

It is best to eat all vegetables and fruits immediately after harvesting them, once they are fully ripe. This is particularly true for tomatoes, which are very cooling and can worsen some disorders, such as rheumatism. Taken in moderate amounts, they are useful for circulatory problems.

Radishes have cooling qualities, in spite of their burning taste. They are recommended for certain disorders but can aggravate others, such as coughs and colds.

Potatoes tend to worsen *pegen* and kidney disorders, when eaten in excess, because of their cooling qualities. In such cases, this can be counter-balanced by frying them and adding spices, such as cardamom, nutmeg, and pepper, that make them more warming and lighter. Potato peels are difficult to digest. Individuals with weight problems are advised to limit their consumption of potatoes.

Aniseed and fennel stimulate the production of milk in new mothers. Parsley has the opposite effect.

Fruits are not cited as a separate category in the medical texts; however, they are described in teachings of Tibetan medicine. Fruits are sweet and sour. It is important to eat them well-ripened so they are lighter, warming and sweet, while green fruits are heavy and sour. Certain fruits, such as bananas, papayas, and mangoes, are naturally warming and are useful to improve digestion. Apples and pears affect the energies less than most other fruits. It is preferable to eat grapefruit after bread and honey or other cereal-based food, due to its acidity. Pomegranates are especially good for health and are an important component of some Tibetan remedies. Moreover, laboratory studies have shown that pomegranates contain substances that slow down and even stop the growth of cancerous cells (Sharma, McClees and Afaq, 2017).

Any excess of the sweet or sour quality can be harmful. However, the sugar of fruits possesses a heating effect that is absent in refined sugar. It is better to eat fruits, especially melon, in the absence of other food. If eaten with a meal, fruit should be eaten at the beginning, so it does not stay long enough in the stomach to start to ferment.

Most fruits and vegetables that are not organic contain dangerous pesticides, herbicides, and other chemicals that are factors in the development of cancer, neurological diseases, and reduced fertility. Some foods have been found to contain higher levels than others. These include: strawberries, nectarines, apples, grapes, peaches, cherries, pears, tomatoes, and peppers, but there are many others. In order to remove the harmful chemicals, fruits and vegetables can be soaked several minutes in a solution of sodium bicarbonate (a small spoon for two cups of water) and then rinsed.

Health-wise, the best chocolate is the dark variety. However, all chocolate is harmful in the case of migraines, in which case, it is advised to eat bitter food to counter the excess heat.

Patients with itchy rashes should avoid garlic, mangoes, bananas, and especially alcohol. Garlic is particularly bad for persons with acne and other skin disorders.

Eggs are not mentioned in the medical texts, but Jacques Haesaert cited Dr. N. T. Dingghang's teachings, "They are considered to be the essence of birds. Their importance is very great at the vital level. They ameliorate the aura and general appearance of the body, as well as increasing sperm." Consumption of fresh, organic eggs increases a person's vital force. However, an excess of eggs, especially when boiled, tends to decrease body heat and can affect digestion.

Liquids regulate thirst and the three energies. Water, milk, beer, and other alcoholic beverages are mentioned the most frequently in medical texts.

Milk is sweet, oily, and heavy. It is generally beneficial, except in the case of *pegen* disorders—such as kidney problems, coughing, and colds, because of its heaviness and cooling power. It is an essential food, like eggs, because it increases vitality. However, it is advised to avoid drinking cold milk. Concentrated milk with added sugar has the cooling qualities of refined sugar added to that of the milk. Mixed with water, milk is more easily digested than without. Fat-free milk is hard to digest.

It cannot be stressed enough how extremely beneficial it is for mothers to breast-feed their babies. No substitute can even come close to this ideal food. There are enormous advantages for the mother as well as the baby. Moreover, in many cases, a sick baby can be treated by treating the mother.

Milk is a good example of how the quality of substances depends on the species of the animal. Goat's milk is lighter and more refreshing than cow's milk. Sheep's milk is heavier and oilier. Horse and donkey milk have other qualities still.

Fresh white and yellow cheeses have very different properties than old ones such as blue cheese. Fresh cheeses have softening and heavy qualities and combat *lung* disorders. Old, strong-smelling cheeses should be avoided in the case of migraines, cancer, eczema, and certain other disorders.

There are seven types of water mentioned in the medical texts: rainwater, melted snow, river water, mineral spring water, well water, sea water, and forest water. Each has specific qualities. Seawater or salt water from lakes cannot, of course, be consumed but it is useful for therapeutic baths. As described above, it is not favorable, in general, to drink cold water. However, it can combat the influence of alcohol, stupor, nausea, or dizziness. Boiling water gives it a lighter quality.

Alcohol is harmful for patients with many types of disorders. There are, however, a few specific cases when it can be beneficial in small quantities. The qualities of beer are roughness and force. It can aid digestion, help a person to sleep. Young wines are acidic and not recommended. All alcoholic beverages have harmful effects if drunk in excess, also causing one to lose their self-control. Long-term excessive consumption of alcohol weakens the liver and lungs as well as the vitality of the body, affecting vision, the brain, and sometimes the heart. Alcohol is very harmful for the developing fetus in the womb.

Moreover, it has also been shown to be harmful in every type of cancer studied in clinical tests.

Black tea is stimulating due to its warming, astringent, and coarse qualities. Coffee is warming and stimulating, but also possesses very serious undesirable effects. Tibetan physicians consider that coffee intake should be limited because it affects blood and creates ocular disorders by affecting certain powers of the liver. They consider this to be a major cause of ocular disorders in the West. These disorders are much rarer among Tibetans who never drink coffee. They drink only tea, whose effects are very different.

Various types of salt, such as sea salt, rock salt, saltpeter, and ammonium salt are used for consumption or in medicines. Table salt has warming qualities and, therefore, facilitates digestion.

Hot-tasting spices, such as pepper and chilli, stimulate the appetite, facilitate digestion, and are warming. Eaten in excess, they cause haemorrhoids. This is often observed in India. Spices such as nutmeg, ginger, cardamom, clove, and cumin are very useful in the case of *cold* disorders, as food and in other therapies. They generally open the appetite, aid digestion, and give a pleasant taste to food. Saffron has recently been found to have profound benefits on age-related macular degeneration and retinitis pigmentosa (Ramírez et al., 2020; Broadhead et al., 2018).

White sugar is cooling, gives a pleasant taste, and increases the person's desire for more sweet foods. It is harmful for overweight people. In general, it is much better to use honey instead of sugar.

Eating according to the seasons

The following advice is rarely heard in Western culture:

It is better to considerably modify our food choices when we pass from one season to another. In our modern world, it is possible to find out-of-season foods at any time, but fruits and vegetables are picked and transported long before they are ripe, and one should limit eating them.

According to the specific dominant energy of each season, the following are the best foods to eat and those to be avoided:

- In spring: bitter, spicy, and some sour foods work to prevent cold *pegen* disorders from arising. Examples of good choices include stews and boiled water with honey. Nature gives us asparagus in the spring and this is the time to eat it.
- In summer: protein in the form of goat cheese and raw tofu, and some salads are recommended. In-season fruits and vegetables, wholegrains rather than white cereals, and sufficient quantities of water are recommended. Foods to be limited are animal fat and warming foods, such as meat casseroles with hot spices.
- In autumn: foods fostering reasonable amounts of internal heat, such as soups, fresh butter, apples, aubergine, carrots, parsnips, and butternut squash are recommended while cooling foods are not. *Triba* accumulates at the end of summer; therefore, this is the moment to avoid very warming foods. This includes fatty or fried, heavy foods, abundant spices, and alcohol. Instead, fat-absorbing food like cauliflower and radishes are very good.
- In winter: sweet, sour, and salty tastes are recommended. It is preferable to eat food that is easy to digest, such as white bread and rice rather than whole grains. White bread, however, is not recommended for overweight individuals, as discussed above. Warming foods, spices, garlic, onions, root vegetables, soups, especially bone-marrow soup, are especially good to eat. More protein is recommended in the winter season. The most harmful foods in winter are tomatoes, cucumbers, refined sugar, raw green vegetables, and excesses of cold, raw food, in general.

BEHAVIOR AND NUTRITION   77

Toxic foods and bad combinations

Certain combinations of substances that are individually non-toxic make up one category of poisons. In Tibetan medicine, three types of poisons are described: natural poisons present in plants, minerals, and animals; manufactured poisons; and two types of food poisons that are formed by rotting food or are formed inside the body through combinations of substances that are non-toxic alone.

The following are examples of toxic combinations and foods that should be avoided:

- Milk generally combines poorly with all acidic foods including fruits, acidic vegetables, and alcohol. It also combines poorly with fish or nuts.
- Burned eggs are poison.
- Tomatoes acidify when combined with starches. This is why the consumption of pasta with tomato sauce is not recommended. However, once again, this is general information, and indeed, this combination does not seem to negatively affect most Italians!
- Honey mixed with old butter or oil is poison.
- Coffee mixed with ice cream indirectly creates poisons from undigested food, resulting from increased *lung* in the stomach.
- Yogurt with fruit, especially certain types, is very harmful. The combination of yogurt plus banana, nuts, or apple is extremely bad, especially for women, causing menstrual problems, such as irregularity or too heavy or too little bleeding.
- The combination of yogurt with sugar and certain vegetables can lead to arthritis. Chicken or peas with yogurt should also be avoided.
- It is better to avoid non-organic chicken because of hormone treatments given to the animals and consequences of bad treatment of the animals.

- Rice with sugar or honey is harmful for the sinuses. It can provoke growth of bacteria and parasites in the body due to the excess *pegen* produced.
- A mixture of sugary food with sour and raw food can be harmful.
- The combination of eggs and fish is a poison.
- Peaches mixed with other fruits should be avoided.
- Fried mushrooms in general, and particularly in mustard oil, are poisons.
- The combination of tobacco with strong coffee and lemon juice is very harmful for the energy of the lungs.
- Frequent consumption of cold water or cold milk at the same time as orange juice creates *lung* disorders and conditions for asthma.
- Fried or roasted foods mixed with sour foods such as lemon and vinegar can lead to an infection of the wisdom teeth.
- An excess of sour and raw foods affects the energies of the spleen and affect both lymph and blood.
- Frequent absorption of alcohol with cheese weakens the vitality of the lungs and leads to pulmonary disease. This, however, contradicts common practice in France, where the consumption of cheese together with red wine is widespread. It is, therefore, worth considering if a person suffers from such disorders.

Diets and fasting

A strict limitation of food consumption should not be taken lightly. Each person must be considered individually. If fasting is recommended by a doctor, they will explain how to gradually reduce food intake, how many days to fast, and how to gradually restart eating. In general, the person's physical and mental state, lifestyle and environment should be taken into consideration. Larger amounts of food than usual are even recommended in the case of excess of the light *lung* energy, for those who are weak and elderly, for disorders of the lungs, and insomnia. Likewise, more highly nutritious foods are also beneficial after substantial loss of blood by haemorrhage or excessive menstruation, after childbirth, after excessive sexual relations, and in the spring when the body is weakened and *lung* increases.

Of course, there are cases where food intake should be limited, and not just in the case of obesity. For example, an overly-nutritious diet is harmful in the case of ulcers, mental torpor, excessive urination, and *pegen* disorders.

CHAPTER 7

What is disease, disorder?

When we are sick, most people have a tendency to say "I'm sick", and not "My body is sick". We are thus identifying ourselves as our body, which makes it very difficult to eliminate negative thoughts. If we understand that this disease is not *me*, it is easier to put things in perspective. It is very beneficial to be able to say that I am not my cancer, my flu, I am me and I just happen to have this sickness, but it does not define me.

Sickness is a warning sign, telling us to make changes, so we should try to understand the message and find the positive side of having the disease and especially, to understand its origin.

Teachings on disease are divided into seven parts: primary causes of disease, contributing causes, ways that disease appears, localization of disorders of the three energies, disease characteristics, classification of disease, and individual subjects.

Disease is defined as an unbalanced state, resulting from specific causes and conditions. When one of the subtle energies is too strong or too weak, the resulting imbalance between them always causes disorders. The affected energy leaves its normal localization and goes to where another energy is usually localized and physical symptoms appear. The corporal constituents are affected and subsequently malfunction, which in turn modifies the three impurities. Tibetans use an analogy with the rain to simply explain the phenomenon: Clouds accumulate in the sky. If they meet appropriate conditions, they are transformed into rain, just as disease manifests under certain conditions that have accumulated.

Buddhists also consider physical disease in a spiritual sense, resulting from the three poisons of the mind: desire/attachment, hatred/anger, and ignorance, which causes the other two. These are the primary causes of all illnesses.

There are many other causes and conditions necessary for diseases to manifest. These include:

- wrong proportions of the five elements
- inappropriate behavior
- food, drugs, alcohol, or too little or too much activity
- poor food choices
- emotional shock
- blockage of the movement of one of the energies
- ripening of karma
- spirit intervention
- physical wounds

There are three characteristics of diseases: increase, decrease, and disturbance of the subtle energies; corporal constituents; and impurities. The following are examples of disorders that arise after an increase or decrease in one of the energies:

Increases in *lung* can result in dryness of the body, a bluish complexion, attraction to heat, constipation, and difficulty in sleeping.

Increases in *triba* can cause yellowing of the skin and eyes, excess hunger and thirst, fever, and diarrhea.

Increases in *pegen* can result in a decrease in body heat, digestive difficulties, and heaviness in the body.

Decreases in *lung* cause a lack of energy, mental confusion.

Decreases in *triba* reduce body heat and skin color.

Decreases in *pegen* reduce body fluids.

CHAPTER 8

Classes of diseases

Tibetan medicine is based on an elaborate system of classification, with many criteria; the sex and age of the person, the state of subtle energies, the affected organ functions, and symptoms. Disorders are classified as "cold" or "hot" diseases, which are, therefore, treated with appropriate warming or cooling nutrition and behavior. Without going into detail, some categories of disease are presented here so the reader can appreciate the complexity of this medical knowledge. Eighty-four thousand disorders are described in the medical texts.

There are five classes of disease according to the type of patient; those affecting men, women, children, or the elderly, and general diseases that affect all four groups. Those related to the elderly are not really distinct types, but are generally related to some type of degeneration. Treatment is given to stop the progression of the disease and regenerate the patient's vitality.

The diseases in the above categories are further divided into four sub-categories; diseases of the subtle energies, karmic diseases, psychiatric diseases, and miscellaneous diseases.

The disorders of each energy type have principal locations; *lung* diseases are generally situated in the lower portion of the stomach, intestines, colon, hip joints, bones, heart, and sense organs; *triba* diseases concern the middle portion of the stomach and small intestines, the navel, liver, eyes, blood, sweat, chyle, lymph, and skin; *pegen* diseases affect the upper portion of the stomach, nose, tongue, chest and head, chyle, flesh, fat, marrow, regenerative fluid, excrement, and urine.

Wounds are caused by internal factors or external elements. Internal disorders in this category include outgrowths of flesh on the skin and wounds in the solid and hollow organs, both of which can become tumors, if not treated.

In the Tibetan medical system, the term "fevers" as opposed to "fever" is used because of the numerous characteristics of different kinds of fever. It is important to be aware that diverse types of fever exist because they cannot all be treated in the same way. The category of fevers and inflammation includes fevers that are unripe, increasing, empty, hidden, chronic, or turbid. Only doctors highly skilled in taking the pulse can distinguish between each of these disorders. Observing high temperature is not sufficient to properly diagnose and treat "fever". Wrong diagnosis and inappropriate treatment of certain fevers can cause the condition to deteriorate further. Tibetan physicians do not always act to quickly reduce the fever, but may instead prescribe medicine to *ripen* the fever, to prevent other disorders arising in the body.

Tibetan medicine also classifies disorders into categories of "diverse diseases", according to other criteria. These include chronic disorders, internal or external diseases, and difficult diseases—characterized by the emergence of a new disorder before the previous one has been healed.

Cancer is not mentioned in the medical texts, as such. However, there are eight types of tumors in the category of chronic disorders.

Many types of poisoning are described, including those by manufactured poisons, rotting food, natural poisons, spirits, highly toxic plants, spiders, scorpions, insects, snakes, and poisoning due to bad food combinations.

Detailed information about diseases and their Tibetan names can be found in Jacques Haesaert's teachings.

CHAPTER 9

Invisible powers and spirits

There are societies and healing traditions in all parts of the world, including Europe, that have accepted the existence of spirits and invisible powers, capable of affecting our health. According to Tibetan medicine, ailments, such as certain sense disorders, paralysis, cancers, epilepsy, and mental illnesses, cannot be cured by ordinary coarse treatments since they arise from subtle causes.

The role of spirits in certain diseases seems to be one of the most difficult to understand, although we are all familiar with stories of possession by spirits, at least through documentaries and movies. Anyone familiar with the Bible has probably read passages concerning demons and other spirits. These include writings in the books of Mark, First Corinthians, Ephesians, and Matthew, notably this quote from Mark 9: 14–29, "… and he foamed, and gnashed with his teeth, and pined away … and when he saw Him, straightway the spirit tare him; and he fell on the ground, and wallowed foaming. … You dumb and deaf spirit, I charge you, to come out of him, and enter no more into him. … And the spirit cried and rent him sore, and came out of him…".

The Catholic church has priests who are exorcists and perform rituals, even to this day. Ange Rodriguez, official exorcist of the Lyon, France diocese for ten years, said in an interview that approximately 500 people come to see him every year in search of exorcism. He continued, "Human beings are capable of great things, but why do we always end up doing terrible things, like mass assassinations like the ones we are seeing now? I honestly think that all the political, economic decisions that hurt people are motivated by demons. Those bad spirits are pushing us to take these decisions."

Possession is promoted by the practice of communicating with spirits, which attracts these types of beings who are trying to continue their terrestrial activities. Tibetan doctors strongly advise people not to undertake such practices. Jacques Haesaert wrote, "Tibetans consider this practice to be egotistical, because we only think about prolonging the contact with a parent or another being without asking if this contact is beneficial, sometimes even just using this contact to gain something for ourselves. It is also criminal because we can create great damage to other humans by letting spirits work though them, and we become responsible for the harm that the spirits do. Moreover, when we try to contact them, we increase the force attracting them to this plane of existence, invariably resulting in an increase in their suffering because the particularity of these spirits, as we have seen, is to never be satisfied and be eternally frustrated. We should instead pray to help them liberate themselves from the desire that prevents them from reaching superior planes of existence."

The spirit realm is vast and varied. The first category of spirits includes the gods or governors called *sadak*. They are found everywhere. There are *sadak* guardians of places, such as ponds, and also *sadak* guardians of our harmony and our possessions. If someone tries to take or damage something, consciously or not, they automatically attract the reaction of the *sadak*, by virtue of the law that states that a person cannot harm someone without harming himself.

Jacques Haesaert told his students the story of a young man who came to ask for his help because his body had suddenly developed a strong fetid odor. This strong smell could not be eliminated by extensive, repetitive washing or deodorants. It was repelling his friends and acquaintances and was ruining his life. Jacques listened to him attentively in order to understand what could have triggered this strange condition. After a long discussion, he asked him to take a moment to try to remember exactly when the problem began, and if he could associate it with any time he had spent outside, near a body of water, for example, stagnant water in a woods. After some thought, the young man, said yes, he had taken a walk in the countryside and there was a pond there. Then Jacques asked if he remembers urinating in a particular place that day. The young man said, "Yes, I remember that I pissed into the pond". Jacques was very happy because he had found the remedy for the problem. He said that the young man, by urinating into the pond, had surely angered the *sadak* of the pond, who then bestowed the fetid odor on him. There was no chemical, no physical way of eliminating the problem except to return to that place and sincerely ask forgiveness to this invisible being for offending him. The young man did as Jacques suggested, and immediately the odor disappeared.

Another class of spirits is that of the "hungry ghosts" (*pretas*, in Sanskrit). The cause for rebirth as a hungry ghost is a constant search for material possessions or spiritual powers. After death, this energy creates a subtle mental body similar to the dream state, and this being tries to continue living as before, for example, smoking a cigarette. The hungry ghost is attracted to pleasant experiences of the human plane and becomes frustrated because he cannot satisfy his desires. The *preta* may try to communicate with people he knew, in vain, because he is convinced that he has a normal body, just as we are persuaded that we are having real experiences with our physical body while dreaming.

The most harmful category of spirits is that of the *demons*, because they seek evil. These subtle beings, called *narak*, reside in hell, but can have contact with certain humans. The causes of reincarnation in the hell realm include evil acts, such as killing. There is also another category of internal demons, which are the fruits of our mental creation. While *sadak* work to protect our harmony and peace, demons do the opposite. This explains our everlasting combat between the forces of good and evil.

Babies and young children are particularly prone to possession and should be protected. Tibetans take this very seriously. Certain spiritual practices and contact with very negative people and places with heavy histories of killing and suffering are systematically avoided. Tibetan children wear amulets and receive blessings for protection.

Although it is certainly difficult for many to understand a connection between a disease, such as a type of skin disorder or schizophrenia and spirits, this can encourage us to reflect a little before dismissing the possibility of possession.

CHAPTER 10

Symptoms and diagnosis

Symptoms

During a consultation with a Tibetan doctor, the patient gives important information about their symptoms, activities, work, family situation, nutrition, emotions, important events in their life, and their medical history. The way that they respond to questioning by the doctor also provides useful information about their mental state. The patient may respond, for example, with surprise, anger, embarrassment, or with short or lengthy answers.

In all, there are twenty-nine symptoms of *lung* conditions. Among these are yawning, shivering, sighing, dizziness, shooting pains, dulling of the senses, and pain in the back and joints. One may hear buzzing or other sounds in the ears, or feel cold. In individuals with *lung* disorders, sadness, anxiety, and nervousness are often found. Typical *lung* disorders include arrhythmia, tachycardia, lack of oxygen, impotency, menstrual problems, and insomnia. The symptoms are most evident when the patient is hungry. The physician will detect a pulse that is "elastic", meaning that when they press strongly, it disappears, and then immediately reappears when the pressure is removed. The patient's urine is clear, abundant, bluish, and foamy. A rough, dry, and red tongue and an astringent taste in the mouth are also symptoms.

Among the symptoms of a *triba* disorder are a pale-yellow tongue with a thick coating and a bitter taste in the mouth. The person's eyes and complexion may be yellowish. They may have fever and sweating. Sometimes, the patient shows signs of aggressiveness. *Triba* disorders include heart attack, hepatitis, migraine, thyroid problems, high blood pressure, and skin disorders.

Symptoms of *pegen* disorders include a weak, barely perceptible pulse and pale, odorless, and vaporless urine with small bubbles. The tongue has a pale coating. The patient often feels heaviness and bloating in the stomach and a lack of strength. They may also not be able to taste food. They may have pale skin and swollen eyes and cheeks, abundant mucus, excessive drowsiness, confused memory, and an increase in body weight. *Pegen* disorders include obesity and diabetes.

Diagnostic techniques

Observation and questioning

General diagnoses are made by interrogating and observing the patient, which enables the physician to decern how the patient is feeling, what they are experiencing, and why they requested a consultation. In the medical tantras, observation of urine and the tongue is mentioned, but in practice, the skin complexion, eyes, ears, nails, the aura of the patient, their posture, gait, and flexibility are also observed.

The way the patient speaks is also revealing; whether they speak willingly or not, slowly or quickly, loudly or softly. The sound of their voice is also noted. A high-pitched sound is a sign of excess *triba*, a hoarse and weak sound, *pegen*, and low and cavernous sound, *lung*.

Diagnostic techniques used in Tibetan medicine could be extremely useful for Western doctors. Particularly interesting for pediatricians are the observation of the veins in babies' and small children's ears, observation of the mother's milk, and the interpretation of the baby's crying.

Consultations last at least forty-five minutes and always include questioning the patient extensively about their usual way of eating and recent food choices, habitual behavior, recent actions and experiences, work, sleep patterns, emotions, symptoms, current medication, and their moral stance. The medical history for the patient and their family also is noted. Attentively listening to the patient and taking careful consideration of what they have to say is an important part of the doctor's ethical practice. This patient-physician dialogue establishes a climate of confidence that is indispensable for the patient's healing.

The art of palpation includes pulse diagnosis and checking for painful areas, which indicate where the illness is located. Diagnosis by palpation of such regions as the abdomen includes observation of the patient's reaction to it. Touching each painful area indicates the state of the related organs. There are important points along the vertebrae and on the head.

Taking of the pulse is extremely important and is always used for diagnosis. The doctor's fingers are indeed weapons against disease, for by skillfully taking a patient's pulses, the doctor can evaluate the health of each internal organ.

I cite some examples of specific diagnoses based on the pulse explained by Jacques Haesaert to show the depth of the information acquired:

"In the case of dysentery, *Truk-tse*, the pulse is thick and rapid; the sex pulse is particularly rapid. In the case of skin disease, of which there are sixty-four principal types, the pulse is usually trembling. In the case of leprosy, the pulse is changing in quality. The pulse of the patient with an infectious and contagious disease is rapid but weak. In the case of tuberculosis, two types of pulses are felt in the same place, with equal force. When there is sudden pain in part of the body, the pulse has abrupt palpitations; pain in the stomach or intestines causes the pulse to be rapid and firm. In the case of external wounds, there are two pulses: one strong and one thin. If the wounds are internal, the pulse shivers and gives the impression of trying to extend outwards. When there is accumulation of matter, such as pus, the pulse is felt as short pulsations, which is one of the twelve pulses. In the case of accumulation of water, the pulse is drifting and firm, which is also one of the twelve pulses. Diseases caused by pathogens such as viruses are indicated by a flat and oscillating pulse. ..."

We see thus that the art of taking the pulse is extremely complex and that the information available to the physician is considerable. Twelve major pulses are described and thirteen sections on pulses are found in the texts. Long studies are required to master the taking and interpretation of each of the major pulses. The Tibetan system is based on, but is not identical to, the Chinese system.

Observation of the zones of the eyes in order to check the functioning of the organs is standard diagnostic technique in Tibetan medicine. Two examples of the information obtained are; the rhythm of contraction of the pupils—can indicate a *lung* disorder; the condition of the white of the eye and the iris—can indicate the state of the corporeal constituents.

Observation of the tongue's color, texture, thickness, and an eventual coating enables the physician to identify the patient's energetic state. In a *lung* disorder, the tongue is red, rough, and dry. In the case of a *pegen* disorder, it is soft, whitish, and humid. In a *triba* disorder, the tongue is yellowish, especially in the middle, and has a thick coating. Disorders of more than one subtle energy can also be diagnosed.

Analysis of the urine includes observing the color, odor, quantity, taste, the presence of blood, thickness, sediment, bubbles, the formation of vapor, and changes in these parameters over time. The physician learns which subtle energy is affected and if the disorder is *cold* or *hot*, whether due to a poison or spirit attack, and so on. A large quantity of urine indicates a *hot* disorder, while a small quantity indicates a *cold* disorder. There are also particular signs of death that can be detected by noting the qualities, quantities, and changes in the urine.

Urine contains two types of sediments, *trima* and *kuya*. *Trima* is the result of the melting of fat in the body and is indicative of a *triba* disorder, such as fever or inflammation. Like fat, it is light and floats on the surface of the urine. *Kuya* is heavier and can be either under the *trima*, in the middle of the urine, or at the bottom, like sand.

Normal urine usually has a pale yellow color, which can vary, however, because of the influence of food. The color, vapor, and odor are observed while the urine is warm. The abundance, form, size, and time needed for the bubbles to disappear after vigorously stirring the urine gives more information about which of the three energies, *lung*, *triba*, or *pegen* is dominant or less prevalent and indicate which organ may be affected. In the case of possession by spirits, they also indicate which type of spirit is affecting the patient.

Diagnosis of disease in children and babies is difficult as they are unable to describe what is wrong and clearly indicate what hurts. Observation of the child's face, the color of their skin and the child's movements give useful indications.

An easy and very useful diagnostic method that is not used in Western medicine is the systematic observation of the mother's milk when the baby is sick. This diagnosis is based on the fact that many childhood ailments are due to the mother's milk, especially during the period when the baby is nourished solely by breastfeeding. The physician observes the color, clarity, thickness, and the taste of the milk. The form and consistency of the milk are then observed after pouring part of it into a glass of water, as illustrated in Figure 10.

Among the information that can be gathered is which subtle energy is affected. When the mother has a *lung* disorder, her milk is foamy, dry, and has a bad taste. In a *triba* disorder, the milk may be bluish, yellowish, or dark, and have a bad odor. In *pegen* disorders, the milk is very thick and heavy.

According to what the doctor observes, they will treat the mother to improve the quality of her milk. The baby is then also treated by giving medicine to the mother. Nursing babies is considered fundamental for the good health of the baby and the mother and is obviously indispensable for this treatment.

DIAGNOSIS USING MATERNAL MILK PUT INTO A GLASS OF WATER

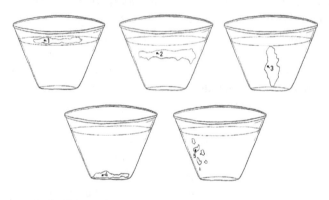

1 - MILK STAYS ON THE SURFACE
THE ILLNESS IS NOT SERIOUS
AND A DOCTOR IS NOT NEEDED

2 - MILK STAYS IN THE MIDDLE
THE ILLNESS IS NOT SERIOUS
BUT A TREATMENT IS NECESSARY

3 - MILK STAYS VERTICAL (PILLAR)
SIGN OF DEATH (VERY SERIOUS AFFLICTION)

4 - MILK STAYS ON THE BOTTOM
VERY SERIOUS AILMENT (DANGEROUS)

5 - MILK FORMS SEPARATE LUMPS
ILLNESS CAUSED BY SPIRITS

Figure 10. Observation of maternal milk in a glass of water.

Observation of veins in the ears of babies and small children is particularly important, as they are unable to describe their discomfort. One enormous advantage of such techniques is that the information is already present, without the need for lengthy and expensive laboratory tests. The ear is divided into three regions, corresponding to the three parts of the body. Specific parts of the ears and their correspondence to organs or vessels are shown in Jacques Haesaert's diagram in Figure 11. He explains how to make the diagnosis as follows; "The posterior side of the ear is observed with the patient's back to the light, so three veins are visible: one extends up, one extends horizontally in the middle part of the ear, and the third one extends downwards. These veins should be red like a rabbit's blood, without branches, and rounded in form so they have no angles. Observation of their colors and form indicate the type of affliction, while the places they are situated indicate which organs are affected".

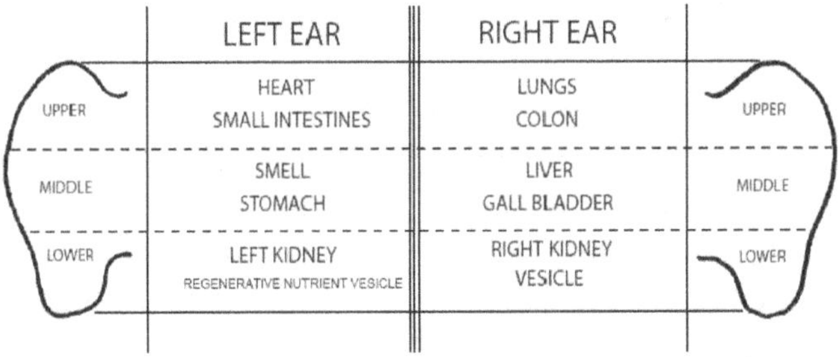

	LEFT EAR	RIGHT EAR	
UPPER	HEART SMALL INTESTINES	LUNGS COLON	UPPER
MIDDLE	SMELL STOMACH	LIVER GALL BLADDER	MIDDLE
LOWER	LEFT KIDNEY REGENERATIVE NUTRIENT VESICLE	RIGHT KIDNEY VESICLE	LOWER

DIVISION OF THE EARS IN FUNCTION OF THE ORGANS, FOR THE DIAGNOSIS BY OBSERVATION OF THE VEINS. (THIS FIGURE IS ONLY VALID FOR A BOY. FOR A GIRL, THE LUNGS AND COLON ARE ON THE LEFT AND THE HEART AND SMALL INTESTINES ARE ON THE RIGHT).

Figure 11. Correspondence of the zones of the ears and organs.

Examples of how veins in various zones of the ears indicate specific diseases are shown in Jacques Haesaert' diagram in Figure 12.

If the color of the veins is:

- bluish, there is a *lung* disorder in the organ corresponding to their location
- yellowish, there is a *triba* disorder
- whitish, there is a *pegen* disorder

LEFT EAR				
UPPER	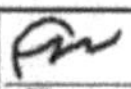	CARDIAC FEVER	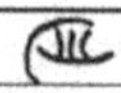	GYE-TSHE * VERY HIGH CARDIAC FEVER
	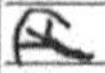	SINUSITIS		
	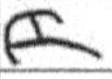	MALE SPIRIT IN THE HEART	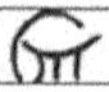	GYE-TSHE : IN THE SMALL INTESTINE
MIDDLE				
LOWER	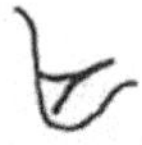	NAGA IN THE KIDNEYS (SPIRITS)	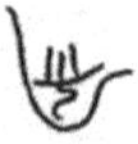	GYE-TSHE : IN THE KIDNEYS

RIGHT EAR				
UPPER	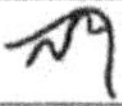	FEVER IN LUNGS	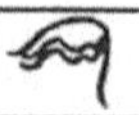	LEAK OF VITAL ENERGY "LA"
	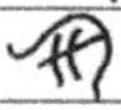	GYE-TSHE : IN LUNGS	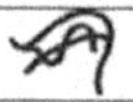	LEAK OF "LA" MORE DANGER OF DEATH
MIDDLE	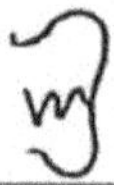	HEPATIC FEVER	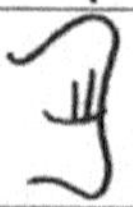	GYE-TSHE : IN THE LIVER
LOWER				

SIGNS OF DISEASE IN VEINS

AS FOR FIGURE 44, THE SIGNS OF THE UPPER PART OF THE EAR MUST BE INVERSED
FOR A GIRL.

* GYE-TSHE IS A HIGH FEVER

Figure 12. Observation of the zones of the ears: signs of disease.

- dark red-brown, a hot disorder is present
- light yellow, a cold disorder is present
- light red, there is a disorder of *blood* energy

Another diagnostic technique is listening to the sound of the child's voice when he or she cries. The mother and the physician can thus identify the type of disorder. Continuing, high-pitched crying is characteristic of *triba* disorders, while long, deep sounds indicate a cold, *pegen* disorder. A muffled or raspy sound reveals a *lung* disorder.

These diagnostic methods are important because pulse diagnosis is extremely difficult due to children's weak heartbeats.

Observation of a patient's hands is often used. The general form of the hand and its size relative to the arms are observed. The hand is divided into three parts; the region of the thumb defined by the lifeline, the rest of the palm, and the fingers. These areas correspond to *pegen*, *triba*, and *lung*, respectively. The fingers give indications about the state of the organs.

The physician observes the color, width, length, depth, and quantity of the lines of the hand. The dominant energy of the patient is thereby determined *pegen* type lines are pale, large, sinuous, and few in number *triba* type lines are yellowish, long, straight, deep, and continuous. *Lung* type lines are dark in color, superficial, numerous, straight, narrow, confused, and superficial.

Astrological diagnosis and detection of spirits

Another technique absent from Western medicine is astrological diagnosis. Specific invisible beings govern astrological houses, and in the case of epilepsy wherein a spirit is implicated, astrological analysis can be useful. Of course, this is only one aspect of epilepsy and different treatments are proposed when the condition arises under different circumstances.

Spirits have no physical existence, for they are made up of only energy and not of the five elements. Therefore, they cannot be seen or heard. Nevertheless, those that affect humans can be detected and the type of spirit can be identified by various methods—including urine examination, pulse diagnosis, dream analysis, and procedures using dice.

CHAPTER 11

What is healing?

Healing is the re-establishment of balance between the three subtle energies and the return to homeostasis and a state of harmony with other beings and within our environment. Subsequently, symptoms will disappear. Part of healing is to develop mental calm. An agitated mind moves in all directions, while a calm mind is limpid, like an undisturbed lake.

If we consider healing on purely the physical or mental level, we are getting only part of the picture; healing is more complex than eliminating symptoms. We can rid the body of a microbe, cut away a tumor, or stop the bleeding, but Tibetans have understood that true healing takes place also on a spiritual level. All of our previous experiences and emotions play a role in our physical and mental state, and this explains why some people cannot be healed. Moreover, if we heal, without eliminating the cause of the disease, it will come back.

We have all heard the saying, "we are what we eat". Here, we go further—we are also what we think, feel, say, do, and experience. No being is independent, except on the conventional level, as we have seen. Realising this, we are able to address disease by treating the person as a whole, and taking into consideration all of these factors.

Spiritual healing

One of the goals of traditional medicine is to increase the healing power in patients. For Tibetans, the spiritual world and spiritual healing are just as real as the physical world. In fact, in the teachings of Tibetan medicine, it is said that there exists a spiritual practice for each of the 84,000 types of suffering. In the cases of diseases where karma is directly responsible, spiritual practices are so important that other treatments are even considered as secondary.

Healing is achieved through psychological and spiritual practices, such as meditation, prayer, visualizations, and the development of compassion and high morality. Transformation is on the level of subtle vital energies and includes elimination, or at least reduction, of negative emotions.

Many Western practitioners are uncomfortable with mixing medicine and spirituality. Nonetheless, more and more is being discovered about psychosomatic origins of disorders and the role of negative emotions in disease. Some persons would like to call spiritual healing a "placebo effect" or consider it to be just positive thinking or good luck. In any case, even if we cannot identify the exact cause of one's healing, what counts is the benefit received! It is always beneficial for us to just keep an open mind. Here, we can think, "Perhaps the prayers did help! Anyway, I am much better!" As already mentioned, it is not necessary to be a Buddhist, or Christian, or Muslim, or whatever, to get the benefits of spiritual practice.

It takes a lot of work for us to be able to open our minds and peel off our old concepts of how things should be. What happens when we discard a lot of what we think we know? We can finally get to the stage of realising that we are not separated from the rest of nature and the universe and that there is a lot more useful knowledge out there, waiting to be learned and applied.

CHAPTER 12

Therapy

A major interest of Tibetan medicine is that a patient is always treated globally, rather than just addressing his or her symptoms. Moreover, the therapist does not always try to eliminate all invading microorganisms. Jacques Haesaert taught, "When we immediately stop all symptoms of disease, and thus all elimination, we transform our body into a vast reservoir of impurities and toxins so that one day, when the saturation point is reached, the slightest incident created by an exterior agent will destroy the fragile equilibrium that was artificially established. It becomes the drop of water that causes the glass to overflow, setting off an eliminatory storm that is absolutely uncontrollable, such as degenerative disease or cancer that often leads to death."

Tibetan medicine offers means of getting to the causes of disease and suffering and suggests ways of eliminating them. The three aspects of the human being—the physical, mental, and spiritual—are taken into account in the four phases of treatment, as well as for diagnosis. The person is always treated as an individual, because what is beneficial for one person may be harmful to another.

There are three categories of treatment described in the third root of the Tree of Medicine: nutrition, behavior, and the medical treatments themselves.

The importance of choosing appropriate nutrition cannot be stressed enough. Unfortunately, getting the correct information is not easy. A lot of false advice, full of generalities about nutrition, circulates on the internet and it is easy to make erroneous conclusions about what are the best choices. Discrimination is necessary and nothing should be blindly accepted. It is taught in Buddhism that even upon hearing teachings of a qualified teacher, neither the person nor his teachings should be accepted without reflection. So, imagine how much care must be taken when getting information from unknown sources on the internet!

Part of therapy is also changing our lifestyle and behavior. This could be to stop smoking or eat more warm food in winter, or anything else. Understanding the disadvantages of our errors can help us strive to eliminate, or at least reduce them. For example, since inappropriate conduct, violent actions, or staying for long periods under the burning sun contribute to *triba* (hot) disorders, a cool environment is beneficial to those with these symptoms. Someone with a *pegen* (cold) disorder feels better in warm places, keeping active by walking and doing other physical exercise.

Treatments

Among the important types of therapy, we find:

- Herbal medicine. The plants are harvested according to strict criteria, prepared, and purified so they can be used as therapy for a variety of disorders. When harvesting the plants, the root systems of the plants are preserved so the plants will continue to grow, respecting the environment. The medicines are complex combinations of twenty or even many more plants.
- Minerals and oligo-elements.
- Highly diluted components that act on a subtle energetic level rather than a chemical level. I recommend reading the

new book by Dr. Jacques Echard, *Remedies of Energy and the Universe*, which includes transcriptions of case histories, for which he obtained amazing results using a new class of homeopathic remedies.

- Essential oils. Much of the knowledge of essential oils comes from ancient Egyptian medicine. There are many indications for their use.
- Application of ointments to the skin in the case of wounds or swelling.
- Moxabustion—the burning of herbal cones just above acupuncture points, to facilitate healing. They are composed of mugwort, a small herb collected in autumn, when it possesses its specific power. Dried powder is prepared, humidified, and shaped into a cone. This moxa is used to treat pain, certain kinds of indigestion, tumors, arthritis, rheumatism, and other disorders.
- Acupuncture is the application of needles, with or without heat, to specific points. There are approximately 1000 points that can be used. Gold, silver, and copper needles of different sizes are used. It is best when practiced on certain days when the body's energy is closest to the surface and not on others. Acupuncture acts on channels that are more subtle than the nervous system. Tibetan acupuncture is slightly different from Chinese acupuncture.
- Application of golden needles to specific acupuncture points. This method is a mixture of moxa and acupuncture. The top of the needle is formed in such a way as to contain a cone of incandescent herbs. The power of the herb and the heat are transmitted by the gold needle. This is, of course, incomprehensible for Western science, because, again here, it is acting on a subtle energetic level. Golden needles are very effective in treating the various forms of epilepsy, mental diseases, and tumors.
- Massage and acupressure. There are many different types of therapeutic massage using various oils and other

components, according to the disorder. Sesame and almond oils are especially good. Massage is particularly advised for the elderly and postpartum women. It is very effective on persons who do not sleep well. In general, the head is massaged first and the feet last. The person's limbs are massaged outward, towards the extremities, in order to expel the disease. For elderly persons and children, massage should be gentle. Massage is best done in a room with moderate lighting, pleasant smells, gentle sounds, and harmonious colors. Massage is generally not used in summer and hot moments of the day. Patients with hot disorders, such as infection, eczema, or fever are not massaged.

- Mineral baths and cold or hot baths containing medicines. Although cold baths are used for certain conditions, it is generally important to keep the body warm, especially the midriff and lower back. Problems of not being able to conceive a child, menstrual and prostate disorders, as well as lower back pain are particularly worsened by an accumulation of cold in this area of the body.
- Blood-letting can be utilized in cases of certain blood disorders, such as poisoning and high blood pressure. It must never be used on patients younger than sixteen years old, pregnant women, those suffering from nervous disorders, or the weak.
- Cauterization of several types.
- Application of hot or cold water, humid towels, and hot or cold stones on the skin.
- Cupping, whereby cups create a vacuum on the patient's skin for a few minutes and eliminate toxins. It is interesting to see that professional and semi-professional athletes have begun to profit more and more from this method. The characteristic round red marks temporarily left on the skin are now often visible on athletes at swimming competitions.
- Laxatives.
- Emetics.

- Curettage and surgical removal. Teachings explain that incisions in the body damage the subtle canals through which the energies circulate. Therefore, surgery is avoided as much as possible.

The following are also used in therapy:

- Meditation on the Medicine Buddha, recitation of mantras, and other spiritual practices.
- Other healing sounds, such as those of singing bowls. Usage of the bowls for healing should be taught by a qualified tantra teacher. Many people now buy bowls but have no training in using them. If one likes the sound of the bowls and does not know really how to get the best healing benefit from them, they can nevertheless be useful, because anyone hearing these pure sounds will feel more relaxed.
- Colors and precious stones. We are all sensitive to the effect of certain colors on our mood. Understanding how they can affect our emotions on a subtle energetic level permits the patient and doctor to use them for healing. For each person, certain colors and gems are more beneficial than others. The best colors for persons with dominant *lung* are green, violet, lapis lazuli blue, and sky blue. Those for dominant *triba* are sky blue, green, white, and dark blue. The best colors for dominant *pegen* are red, brown, dark green and turquoise. Each of the five chakras is associated with a specific color.
- Protective amulets, skins, or other special objects. Their use is widespread in Tibet, Nepal, and Bhutan. They are considered to be especially important for babies and small children, who are more prone to attacks by spirits.
- Astrological indications.

Without understanding that, fundamentally, no one else is to blame for what happens to us, we may feel that an illness happens by chance or that, bad things happen to us because of other people or events, or are even brought upon us by God. We may ask: "Why did this happen to me?" and feel that injustice was done. This type of feeling is very negative because without an answer, it is even harder to bear our pain and long treatments. We may be tempted to change doctors and have more laboratory tests done, while never finishing a treatment. However, understanding that the root source of our troubles is inside and that they are the results of our past actions, we have an explanation and it can be easier to continue the treatments.

The role of the mind in disease is explained as follows. When something happens to us, only our mind decides if we feel enjoyment or suffering. This is why certain persons can accomplish yogic exploits, such as piercing their bodies with needles without feeling pain. The mind has control over the physical body and can thus create ailments and can heal them. Therefore, in the case of a physical disorder directly caused by the mind, a medical treatment can be efficacious only when the mental attitude that created the disorder has changed. For the most part, mental disorders are based on dissatisfaction or frustration, and it is the mind that must be treated. The physical treatment only helps in re-establishing balance in the body, while the mental treatment can totally heal the disease.

Adjusting one's behavior is an integral part of therapy. Repeated errors, especially sexual ones, weaken the body. As we learn to avoid errors, we can develop the discipline to make the right choices according to the situation and the moment. One type of behavior can have opposite effects in certain situations. For example, in some circumstances, frequent warm showers can be very pleasant and they can increase body heat. However, in other cases, exposure to a lot of humidity is harmful. Persons suffering from inflammatory diarrhea, digestive problems, a common cold, or nose or eye disorders should not bathe immediately after meals and should limit showering. Moreover, frequent washing of the head increases hair loss.

We have also seen that bathing is not good for a woman who has just given birth or is menstruating.

An example of well-chosen behavior is frequent application of oil to the body with massage to combat fatigue, effects of aging, and *lung* disorders. Occasional application of oil to the head, feet, and ears gives a feeling of well-being, and increases body heat.

As mentioned above, Tibetan therapy for a sick baby can be of special interest for Western pediatricians. Generally speaking, Tibetans rarely treat a baby without treating the mother. When a baby is sick, instead of substituting the maternal milk with another kind of milk and giving medicines that are difficult for the baby to assimilate, the doctor treats the mother. The medicines given to the mother treat the baby at the same time through her milk, which itself becomes easier to assimilate.

Sometimes, half the medicines are given to the baby and half to the mother. Of course, this is not possible if a mother is not nursing her child.

Diet as therapy

The term "diet" is used here in the sense of strict choices of what a person eats and/or abstains from eating, as well as food quantity. In Tibetan medicine, diet is used with prudence, although physicians do not ignore the purifying effects of a correct diet. They are also conscious of the inconveniences and sometimes very serious problems that arise if the diet is misused. The suppression of natural needs, such as hunger or thirst can seriously perturb the light *lung* wind energy because of the frustration it creates, leading to physical or mental disorders.

Moreover, some chemical drugs and toxic products accumulate in cells; strict food restriction can result in high levels of these toxins being rapidly released into the blood circulation, creating conditions for disorders.

Tibetan medicine uses adjustments of diet in the case of digestive disorders due to over-eating, especially of fatty foods; stiffness in the limbs; some contagious diseases; fevers in general; gonorrhea; stomach wounds; gout; spleen disorders; brain disorders; urinary difficulties; and *pegen* + *triba* combination disorders.

When specific diets are undertaken with good motivation, there is less likelihood that the person becomes frustrated, which sometimes results in consuming even more food than normal, as a reaction to stopping the diet. This, of course, is the worst thing to do when ending fasting. On the contrary, food intake should be slow and progressive.

Nutrition as therapy

"Nutrition" refers to how we use the powers of nutrients to maintain or re-establish an equilibrium in the body. It is, therefore, very important in therapy.

Taste is an extremely important quality of food and medicines, and it is dictated by the specific combinations of the five elements, as follows: A predominance of water produces a sweet taste, fire plus earth produce a sour taste, fire plus water produce a salty taste, fire plus air produce an acrid taste, water plus air produce a bitter taste, and earth plus air produce an astringent taste.

Food and medicine that are earthy in nature are heavy, strong, smooth, and have a strong taste and odor. They are used to combat *lung* disorders. In patients with excess *lung*, patients improve after taking food and medicines with a sweet, sour, or astringent taste, and they worsen on consumption of foods that have a bitter or burning taste. Medicine and food with softening and heavy qualities combat *lung* disorders.

The tastes and odors of food and medicines whose predominant element is water are not pronounced or strong. They lubricate, humidify, and soften the body and combat *triba* disorders.

The patient's state is aggravated by food having a sour, salty, or bitter taste or which give a burning sensation. There are, however, exceptions due to the particular powers of each plant and each substance.

Food and medicines that are watery and earthy in nature are heavy and, therefore, tend to move downwards, with purgative effects. Castor seed oil is a good example of this and is used as a purgative medicine.

The qualities linked to fire are spicy, light, bitter, rough, and oily. Food and medicine dominated by the fire element produce heat in the body, reinforce the corporeal constituents, and combat cold disorders. Patients are, therefore, given sour, salty, or astringent taste food and medicines and are told to avoid sweets. Medicine and food with rough, burning, strong, and light qualities are recommended for *pegen* disorders. Food should be eaten in reasonable quantities and heavy meals should be avoided.

The qualities linked to the air element are light, cold, rough, strong texture, and whitish. Since they are light, they tend to move upwards and may produce emetic effects. Food and medicine dominated by the air element facilitate movement, including the distribution of nutrients in the body, and combat *pegen* and *pegen* + *triba* disorders.

The qualities of space are always present with the other elements, but there are foods and medicines that have space-specific qualities. Domination of space is generally seen as a hollow form. These food and medicines combat disorders of the three energies.

The qualities, and thereby the effects, of plant-derived and animal-derived medicines, vary with the seasons, the climate, the moment of harvesting, conditions of storage, and the method of preparation, as well as astrological influences.

Even though the choice of treatments depends on the person, there are, nevertheless, some general indications that apply to everyone. Patients are advised to vary their food choices and eat natural food without additives and other harmful chemicals, whenever possible. Persons who cannot produce their own food are advised to choose freshly harvested organic food in order to have well-ripened and fruits and vegetables that are free from pesticides, herbicides, and conservatives, some of which are carcinogenic. In order to protect the cardiovascular system, it is recommended to vary the oils that one eats. It is best to favor virgin, cold-pressed olive oil, walnut, and flax-seed oils, and to not exclude butter, which is rich in vitamin E.

In the last few years, research has been generating more and more data related to the effects of food choices on health. The United States National Institute of Health now estimates that 1/3 of cancers are diet-related (Anand et al., 2008).

There are many foods that have been shown to protect against developing cancer, including those making up the Mediterranean diet. Protective foods include turmeric, which contains the active constituent curcumin that increases in efficacy when consumed with black pepper Studies have suggested that cooked tomatoes, red beets, blueberries, garlic, whole wheat, citrus fruits, several types of mushrooms, licorice, chili peppers, figs, flax seeds, papaya, avocados, spinach, cabbage, broccoli, and cauliflower all have protective effects against cancer Thomas, 2009; Zhang, Talalay, Cho and Posner, 1992; Ba et al., 2021; Kim, Yokoyama and Davis, 2014; Otsuki et al., 2010; Shanafelt et al., 2012; Guidelines on diet, nutrition, and cancer prevention: reducing the risk of cancer with healthy food choices and physical activity. The American Cancer Society 1996 Advisory Committee on Diet, Nutrition, and Cancer Prevention, 1996.

It cannot be stressed enough that the following products are not recommended by Tibetan physicians; margarine, animal fat (with the exception of moderate amounts of butter), trans-fatty acids found in refined oils and foods prepared in the U.S.A., refined sugar, excess salt, excess alcohol and coffee, any drink with added sugar (especially soft drinks), ice-cold drinks, commercial yogurt containing sugar and fruit, and anything containing high fructose corn syrup. This last product, which is widely used in the food industry in North America, is very unhealthy; it goes from the stomach directly to the liver and results in fat build-up in the liver.

Certain foods are known to favor the manifestation of specific disorders.

Medicines and other treatments

A characteristic of Tibetan medicines is that they contain many components. As mentioned before, a simple remedy may contain twenty substances and more complex formulae contain as many as seventy ingredients. This certainly explains some of the amazing results of these medicines. The choice of the components is mainly dependent upon potency and taste. Approximately 500 medicinal formulae are currently in common usage.

The many types of remedies used in Tibetan medicine include decoctions, medicinal powders, medicines made from minerals and precious stones, natural herbs, essential oils, suppositories, and medicines added to water for enemas. We find many substances that are not used in Western medicine.

Precious stones, minerals, and metals are also used in therapy for various disorders. Some examples are:

- Gold, which is bitter in taste, is used to treat cases of poisoning.
- Silver is similar in taste and effects to gold. Silver dries and stops the flow of blood.
- Copper has a sweet taste and cooling quality. It dries up pus and heals pulmonary and hepatic inflammation. It is known also in the West to be bactericidal.
- Rubies, emeralds, agate, and rock crystals are all used to treat various disorders, including those provoked by spirits.

- Sapphires help to restore balance of the three energies.
- Turquoise has a healing effect on liver disorders, in general, and is especially prescribed to treat inflammation. It is also used for various degenerative disorders.
- Yellow topaz and smoked quartz help the lungs heal.
- Garnet can be used in the treatment of the small intestine.
- Mercury is first detoxified and then used in association with sulfur. Pills containing mercury may be given as part of the treatment of cancer or other afflictions of the person's vital force. In all cases, it is impossible to heal cancer without restoring this vital force.
- Saltpeter is used to treat urinary disorders.
- Sulfur is used to heal wounds and inflammation of the circulatory system.

Many parts of trees and plants are used in therapy. The most important medicinal trees are sandalwood, which is used for inflammation of the heart or lungs; aloes wood, which also heals cardiac inflammation, and a tree with the name "true lover's knot" that produces a medicinal resin.

There are so many plant remedies, they cannot be listed here. Animal-derived substances are also used in therapy. The reader can refer to Jacques Haesaert's book for more details of treatments.

We have seen that homeopathic remedies are used. Utilization of the Tibetan doctrine of "similarity" also extends to nutrition. For example, in the case of indigestion of a particular food, a soup made with this same ingredient is given as a remedy. To treat indigestion of butter, whey is used. To treat indigestion of beer, the joints of green stems of rice, barley, or other cereal used for the fabrication of the beer are used as a remedy. In this case, yeast soup can also be given.

The doctrine of similarity is also well known in other cultures. A century after Paracelsus, the botanist William Coles wrote that each plant has some attribute that shows the botanist what its use may be. He believed that God had made "herbes for the use of man, and hath given them particular Signatures, whereby a man may read ... the use of them" (Coles, 1656).

It is clear that the doctrine of similarity extends very far into the plant domain, although it has not yet been possible to verify much of the information. Dr. Ama Lobsang Dolma taught that white plants, in general, are useful in the case of *lung* disorders. From this, it can be deduced that yellow plants are beneficial for *triba* disorders, and so on. This is not entirely speculation, because it is said in Tibetan medicine that anywhere a skillful physician travels, they should be capable of using local medicines, by close observation.

It is interesting to note here that Jacques Haesaert had extensive knowledge of botany, as a naturopath in France, before beginning his studies of Tibetan medicine, and was, therefore, able to use local plants as therapy, upon returning to France. He explained that, by observing a plant, it is possible to have an idea of its relationship with the human body. For example, most humid and hairy plants are soothing for the respiratory tract, they are similar to its hairy mucus membranes. Astringent plants such as water avens or creeping cinquefoil have strong structures with dominant earth element, and yellow flowers indicating that they are connected to the air element, and we know from Tibetan medicine that the air and earth elements dominate in plants having an astringent taste."

Let us take another example: the implications of verbena (*Verveine officinale*) on the nervous system. The plant's stems are thin with many branches, reminding one of neuronal fibers. Verbena is especially beneficial for people with *triba* personalities who push themselves because of ambition to a state of great fatigue and need to unwind. It also has anti-inflammatory properties and action on the digestive system. Verbena's main active ingredient has been found to be verbenalin, which confers its effects on the nervous system.

These are just a few examples to illustrate the Tibetan approach to using what nature gives us.

A physician's knowledge of plants is not limited to botanical species but also includes how the individual power of each plant varies according to the terrain, the time of year, and astral influences that affect the plant's power. Moreover, the potential for medical utilization of a plant depends on environmental factors such as sunlight, moonlight, shade, and humidity.

Another important factor concerning the harvesting of medicinal plants is the state of mind of the person who harvests these plants. It is said that a person should have a good motivation to do this work. If not, they should abstain from doing it and let someone else do it. This precept is also valid for the preparation of medicines and for giving them to patients. We are very far away from the motives of the modern pharmaceutical industry!

Decoctions are principally made from six ingredients: *Gentiana barbata*; two ingredients called manu, and letre; and the three fruits: *Terminalia chebula* (black or chebulic myrobalan), *Crataegus sanguinea* (redhaw hawthorn or Siberian hawthorn), and Crataegus pinnatififa (mountain hawthorn).

Common ingredients of medicinal powders include such substances as camphor, white sandalwood, and saffron.

Two frequent methods of treatment are pacification and cleansing. For example, the pacifying treatment for *lung* disorders includes broths and medicinal oils. Decoctions and medicinal powders are given for *triba* disorders. For *pegen* disorders, pills and medicinal powders are used. The second method of treatment includes giving medicine that provokes vomiting or intestinal evacuation, in order to rid the body of the physical causes of the disorder. The methods of cleansing include enemas for *lung* disorders, purgatives for *triba* disorders, and emetics for *pegen* disorders.

There are many methods used to treat disorders of the three energies. It is not possible to go into detail here; however, the following are some other examples:

- For *lung* disorders, treatments include ointments made principally from sesame oil, pills, massages with warm oil, and moxas.
- For *triba* disorders, decoctions and medicinal powders are given. Other methods include induction of perspiration by enveloping the patient in covers.
- For *pegen* disorders, pills and medicinal powders are used. Other methods include massage with warm oil.

CHAPTER 13

Western dogmas absent from Tibetan medicine

Many Western doctors have recently come to realize that systematically killing off the organisms that invade our bodies is not the best approach to treating disease. We have trillions of bacteria in our cells for good reason. It was believed for many years that there were even many more bacteria in our bodies than human cells; however, a study conducted by Milo and Sender (2016) reported that that the number of bacterial and human cells in our body are roughly similar. The correct functioning of our digestive and immune systems is completely dependent on the complex bacterial population in the gut. Systematically killing of invading bacteria destroys the equilibrium of our natural microflora, required for maintaining health. The massive use of antibiotics has also caused devastating proliferation of antibiotic-resistant pathogens that can no longer be eliminated by known treatment. This is another example of how looking at health and disease from a more natural perspective can have long term benefit.

Jacques Haesaert taught us that, "In Tibetan medicine, as in naturopathy, a disease is not an enemy to be eliminated by any means, but rather part of the intelligence of nature, or divine intelligence, that responds to a need we have. This intelligence always provides us with exactly what we need, and only what we need. By observing the manifestations of disease in the body, we can understand what we need and help the disease to accomplish its work instead of preventing it from doing so, as we usually do."

A disease usually manifests as an increase in elimination; stools, perspiration, vomit, pus, which corresponds to a need for the body to purify itself. In certain circumstances, it can, therefore, be extremely harmful to stop these eliminations that should be allowed to proceed. Of course, when excess elimination endangers certain organs, medicines can be used to control it, without completely stopping it.

Likewise, it can be harmful to immediately cool down the body, in the case of some types of fever. In certain circumstances, the best advice is to let the fever take its course, rather than make any attempt to control it using antipyretics.

CHAPTER 14

The Tibetan medicine approach to several common diseases

The following describes some diseases particularly common in the West.

Allergies

Hay fever and allergies are not frequently encountered in Tibet. The apparent causes are substances present in our environment, but the real cause is principally a weakness of the body that induces this hypersensitivity. This disorder is due to poor food choices. Avoiding prepared foods and drinks containing sugar is usually sufficient for eliminating these types of problems. Medicines are given to treat nasal inflammation, sinus infections, and bronchitis.

Asthma

There are five different types of asthma described in the texts. It is either of the allergic type or can be due to a direct internal cause. They are all *pegen* diseases and are due to a decrease in the power of the lungs. *Pegen* produces excess mucus and saliva, feelings of cold and heaviness, and difficulty in breathing. The increase in *pegen* also decreases the heat of *triba*, resulting in poor digestion. The disorder sometimes exists from birth, for karmic reasons, but nutrition is an essential factor in its amelioration or worsening. Certain food combinations, food and beverages that are cold in power and/or temperature, and sour food destroy the power of the lungs. Coffee is also an important negative factor and it can even antagonize the effect of medicines that are given.

Cancer

There are descriptions of various types of tumors in the medical texts, although "cancer" is not a separate category of specific diseases. It is not treated with surgery, chemotherapy, and radiotherapy, although a Tibetan medical doctor would not suggest to a patient that they refrain from their Western medical treatment. Clinical studies undertaken in the United States and elsewhere have shown Tibetan medicine to be safe and to have positive effects on quality of life, disease regression, and remission in patients with cancer. Tibetan medical treatments to reduce the devastating effects of chemotherapy and radiotherapy are very effective. Modification of the patient's diet is always recommended (Bauer-Wu et al., 2014).

The Tibetan medical treatment for cancer is to first break down or dissolve the cancer growth, then pacify the predominant subtle energy involved, reduce inflammation, and then heal the affected organ and the rest of the body.

Prevention is very important. Tibetan medicine teaches that poor choice of lifestyle and feelings of dissatisfaction, as well as toxic chemicals and other forms of pollution, are major factors in the manifestation of cancer. Long term errors in food choices play a role in the development of cysts and nodules into tumors. Too much cold energy accumulates in the body because of inappropriate behavior and cooling food.

Dr. Lobsang Shrestra advises cancer patients to refrain from drinking any alcohol or cold drinks and eating acidic unripe fruits, anything containing vinegar or soy sauce, fermented foods, blue cheeses, kaki, coffee, light green lettuce, strong curry powder, raw onions and garlic, hot chili peppers, pork, non-organic chicken, olives, and frozen food in general. Fruits with "hairs", such as peaches, apricots, and kiwis should be avoided. Alcohol particularly boosts metastases. Turmeric and pomegranates are especially recommended.

Cardiac diseases

The heart is considered to be the king of all the organs. It is a repository of all our positive and negative mental afflictions. Positive mental factors such as happiness, love, and compassion and negative mental factors like anger, hatred, and worry are all based and developed in the heart.

Cardiac disorders are principally caused by mental tension, anxiety, heavy responsibilities, and especially by an excess of foods and drinks that are heating in taste and in quality. There are seven types of heart disease, which are subdivided according to which subtle energies are dominant. The illnesses have similar physical signs and symptoms. Therefore, in order to establish a correct diagnosis, doctors inquire about the case history of the patients and examine the patient's eyes, tongue, urine, and pulse to identify the energy imbalance. The doctor will, for example, observe eyes that are reddish when the nature of the disease is *triba*, pale and watery in the case of *pegen*, and dry and rough in the case of *lung*.

Cataracts

The main causes are liver disorders and impure blood. Long term consumption of sour, acidic foods is a contributing cause. The liver, which is considered to be the principal cause, is treated first, and then surgery can be undertaken. Until surgery could be performed in Tibet under good conditions, the principal treatment consisted of first giving a light decoction to open up body channels, then a medicine containing forty ingredients including iron powder, myrobalan fruits, and saffron was given.

Common cold

Although this disorder is called a "cold", it is, in fact, a hot disorder. Under normal conditions, the skin's pores close in cold weather in order to conserve the body's internal heat. If the cold pushes on the "doors" of the nose in order to enter the body, its meeting with the internal body heat damages the passageways of the nose, which is the door of the *lung* subtle energy. The disorder then spreads throughout the whole system, since *lung* is the energy connecting all the elements of the body. The lungs are especially affected and if the disorder becomes chronic, it can combine with other disorders to which the individual has a high propensity and become a more serious disease.

Depression

This *lung* disorder is considered to be a lack of connection to objects of pleasure. A person who does not experience happiness or suffering is indifferent to the world around him. Without sensations, the person loses his vitality. Not only do they lack compassion for others, they have no compassion for himself, as well. The patient has a fixation on his own problems and believes something outside of themselves is the cause of this suffering. The way for the person to heal is by understanding that it can only come from helping others.

A physician will advise him to change the way they look at their life, to meditate on the good things, such as being born in a secure country with available health care, without war or famine, having relatively good health, having a job that provides a salary, even if it is not their first choice, while so many have no or very little income, and having a family, even if there are tensions that arise, while many others are completely alone. They can then develop compassion and begin to help others.

A depressed person may need to do something about chronic work stress before being well enough to help others. The stress may even have come from doing good deeds beyond his physical capacity and feeling frustrated from not doing more. In these cases, the person needs to be kind to themselves and get the rest that they desperately need. Major lifestyle changes may be required.

In very serious cases of depression, herbal medicines and other treatments, such as moxabustion, are given by the physician.

Diabetes

This is a chronic, *pegen* disease, with excesses of cold and water. Long term inappropriate food choices affect the digestive system so that the liver, gall bladder and spleen, as well as the pancreas, do not function correctly. Cold, sweet and acidic foods should be avoided as well as refined cereals and alcohol. Besides physical treatments, such as massage, acupuncture, and herbal medicines, spiritual practices are encouraged, because again, the influence of karma is very important in this disease.

Diarrhea

There are two principal types of diarrhea—hot and cold. However, the symptoms can be mixed, as in the case of diarrhea due to parasites. Cold diarrhea is usually caused by indigestion due to insufficient *digestive fire*. This disorder tends to become chronic, and the person's vitality slowly diminishes. After eating, some whole pieces of food may be expelled from the body. The patient's corporeal constituents slowly degrade. Weakness of the digestive power is principally due to the consummation of foods that are cold in quality and temperature and that are heavy and without essence. Behavior such as sitting in cold places, having too much contact with water, or having a mental attitude that affects the digestive energy are also important factors in this disorder.

An excess of heat or infection can cause two types of hot diarrhea. It can be provoked by excessively hot environmental conditions, overly warming beverages, or for another reason. This diarrhea is characterized by painful and powerful expulsions and a very rapid loss of vitality. It can be provoked by the combination of a common cold and intestinal disorders.

Drug addiction and alcoholism

There are two principal medicines used to treat drug addiction. The first one causes the patient to become sick if they take a drug. The second medicine calms the *lung* increased by the absorption of alcohol and balances the three subtle energies in order to eliminate the physical base that causes the drug dependence. The permanent need to drink can be eliminated by this medicine, restoring feelings of satisfaction and fighting the tendency to drink.

Epilepsy

There are seventeen types of epilepsy. This disorder has a physical aspect associated with brain damage and a subtle one due to spirit intervention. Physical causes include absorption of contaminated foods, especially pork; inhalation of certain types of smoke; certain acidic food; alcohol; and all other behavior that damages brain power, including trauma. Effective therapy takes both aspects of epilepsy into consideration. According to the type of epilepsy, the treatment includes medicines, acupuncture, the use of heated golden needles, and spiritual practices. Some forms of epilepsy are incurable. Certain astrological influences can affect the crises.

Numerous case histories and testimonials have shown that Tibetan medicine is as effective as pharmaceuticals for controlling crises, but there is insufficient evidence to yet determine whether the use of Tibetan medicine is scientifically sound.

Hypertension

This disorder is characterized by the overheating of *lung* in the blood due to mental or physical causes. Medicines including such plants as *Emblica officinalis* (myrobalan) and *Corydalis hendersonii* are given for at least two or three months for hypertension. Traditional treatment included giving medicine to separate the bad blood from the good, followed by bloodletting, however this is rarely practiced.

Menstrual disorders

In Tibetan medicine, menstrual fluid is not considered to be a waste product, but rather as something vital. It should be sufficient but not over-abundant, and periods should be regular. Disorders are the result of energy imbalance and too much heat or cold in the body. They are caused by either an excess of heat in the blood or by *thursel lung*, the subtle energy that controls downward movements in the lower part of the body. In the first case, medicine is given to cool the blood. In the second case, the disorders are partially the result of too much cold energy, again because of poor choices of behavior and food. There may be an excess, a lack, or irregularities of the menses. Sometimes there is no menstruation because *thursel lung* moves upward. The abdomen swells, the eyes are affected, and the kidneys are painful. The blockage of this *lung*, for example, because of ingestion of excessively sour food, too much sugar or ice cream, provokes the accumulation of water and cold in the abdomen. An absence of periods or excess blood loss may be caused by *thursel lung* or a defect in veins that are not able to contract. In this last case, vasoconstricting medicines are given.

Obesity

This disorder that has become epidemic in many countries is a *pegen* disorder, with its characteristics of cold and heaviness. As well as not getting enough exercise and eating too much of the wrong foods and at the wrong times, other factors are very important causal factors here. Consuming too much cold, raw food and sweet cold drinks disrupt the normal function of the digestive system, in part by altering the make-up of the intestinal flora. Other organs are also affected.

High fructose corn syrup is particularly harmful and is omnipresent in prepared foods in the USA. In addition, excess cold enters the body if one has too much contact with water through daily showers or baths, as in Western society. It has also been clearly shown that these habits favor the growth of undesirable micro-organisms, worsening the disorder, as protective micro-organisms are washed away.

A severely overweight person, likely to eventually develop diabetes, should avoid white bread and other refined cereals, as well as potatoes and sugar. Unripe fruits are acidic and should not be eaten. Some milk is okay if it is warmed first and not ingested directly from the refrigerator.

Paralysis

Damage to brain tissue as the result of an accident or a decrease in the vital force in certain parts of the brain can result in paralysis. Only restoration of this power can improve the patient's condition. Therapy includes modification of the patient's food, specific medicines, and application of moxa, at the correct moment of the treatment. This is very important. Alcohol, tobacco, and coffee are harmful. Certain practices such as massage may be used, but with great prudence if the attack of paralysis was caused by hypertension. As prevention, care should be taken to avoid loss of vital power of the head—this includes washing the head with hot water or diving into cold water without transition when the body is hot, or the contrary, into hot water when the body is cold.

Parasitic diseases

These diseases require long treatments. Extensive training is undertaken to inform populations about prevention, hygiene, and diagnosis. Medicines are given over long periods to not only eliminate the parasites but also to eliminate the poisons created by them.

Rheumatism and arthritis

In modern medicine, rheumatism refers to any disease marked by inflammation and pain in the joints, muscles, or fibrous tissue. Tibetan medicine refers to two types of arthritis: cold and hot. The cold type, which we know as "arthrosis", is characterized by a destruction of bone and cartilage through wear-and-tear. It can become osteoarthritis, with inflammation, over time. Hot arthritis, which includes rheumatoid arthritis and gout, begins as an inflammation. Rheumatoid arthritis is the chronic disease known in Tibet that can affect other body systems, as well as joints.

Once again, it can be stated that a Tibetan doctor knows that long term bad food choices, including too much cold and sour food, as well as too much long-term contact with humidity and cold temperatures lead to cold disorders. These diseases are good examples for which prevention over our lifetime is very effective. The lymphatic disorders at the origin of arthritis are due to poor circulation of fluids through the kidneys and recurring exposure of the middle and lower part of the body to cold temperatures. The cold in the feet can go up to the kidneys, through the bones.

Rheumatism and arthritis are principally treated by moxa, exercise, medicinal baths, and compresses. Herbal medicines can be given against hidden fever in locally inflamed regions in joints, characterized by acute pain. The choice of nutrition is important, and vinegar and foods containing it are particularly harmful, as well as soy sauce and yogurt with sugar. Raw foods, excess salt, milk, and cabbage should be avoided. In the case of hot arthritis, the patient should not drink alcohol. The practice of Tai Chi Chuan is particularly recommended.

Swelling of the body

Swelling can be provoked by excess *pegen* or *pegen* + *lung*. In this last case, the body is swollen not because of *pegen*, but because of *lung*. This swelling occurs in the morning, and it decreases in the evening. When *pegen* is the cause, the body swells in the evening and decreases in the morning. Again, proper nutrition is very important.

CHAPTER 15

Signs, omens, and dreams

In our daily lives, we often have signs or intuition that could be very useful, but we don't perceive them because our numerous physical and mental activities inhibit them. During the dream state, these inhibitions are absent, so we can more clearly contemplate our tendencies to encounter certain situations. The advantage of knowing is not so much to change a situation that is occurring or will occur, but rather to discover its cause. If the law of karma puts us into certain situations where we have a probability of committing certain bad actions, a warning of this coming situation can enable us to momentarily avoid problems. However, it does not prevent this from eventually arising, because the tendency will not have been corrected. What we can do is to profit from the warning in the dream, find the profound cause, and correct it.

It is important to understand, however, that some omens are "consequential" and others are not. It is an art to interpret signs and omens and requires extensive study. A doctor sometimes asks about his patient's dreams because they can be significant when they occur in the second part of the night. Those dreams occurring just before awakening can be significant signs and omens, while those occurring during the first part of sleep are strongly influenced by the events of the day or recent situations and the emotions attached to them.

Many examples of favorable and unfavorable signs have been described in the texts. Among the important signs and omens useful for the doctor are those of distant death, imminent death, uncertain death, and certain death. This helps the doctor to decide if treatment should be continued, or if instead, the family should be notified and palliative care should be given. Uncertain signs of death appear because of illness, so when the illness is treated and the patient is healed, the signs also go away. If the signs subsist after the treatment, they are irreversible and death is certain. It is, however, possible to reverse omens and signs of distant or uncertain death that were given in dreams. Methods include meditation and virtuous practices, such as saving animals that were to be sacrificed.

Everyone dreams, but many people don't remember their dreams. There are methods that can be used to remember dreams. One such method is to remain completely still and focus on remembering our dreams immediately after awakening. Any movement can take away the memory. It is also helpful to think, just before falling asleep, that we want to remember our dreams. There is a very interesting book that teaches how to remember our dreams, The *Tibetan Yogas of Dream and Sleep*, by Tenzin Wangyal Rinpoche (*see* Suggested Reading).

CHAPTER 16

Astrology

Astrology has benefited from widespread interest throughout human history. It has been practiced in all parts of the world and by all the great civilizations. Nevertheless, it is difficult for the rational mind to understand how it can have such remarkable effects upon us.

Tibetan Buddhist teachings describe various methods that guide humans and alleviate their suffering, including systems of divination such as Tibetan astrology and the *Mo* divination system, which gives answers to the questions being asked. *Mo* employs dice and there are books on how to interpret the results. The answers given by the *Mo* are regarded as coming from Manjushri, the Bodhisattva of wisdom. These practices offer practitioners a clear perspective on any given situation, in order to make the best choices in their spiritual and secular lives.

Tibetan astrology is extensively used by physicians. It is very useful for diagnosis, and while it is not part of medicine, strictly speaking, it is, nevertheless, part of the medical training. In fact, the Tibetan medical school in Dharamshala founded by his Holiness the Dalai Lama is called the Tibetan Medical and Astrological Institute, because physicians acquire a profound understanding of astrology, in order to help their patients most appropriately. Likewise, the art of interpreting dreams is not

part of medical studies, strictly speaking, but is also traditionally taught, in view of its profound relevance.

While the positions of the planets do not cause life events,
interpretations can be made because they have an influence on
everything in the universe. Time and place of birth are important factors in a person's health and fortune, and these aspects
are not taken lightly. Tibetans consult astrology for every
major event in a person's life, beginning with birth. The most
favorable astrological moment for birth is chosen, and medicine may be given to speed up or slow down the birth process to
permit the child to be born under the most favorable auspices.

Astrology is used to determine whether a patient can be
healed and, if so, the best date for beginning treatment. There
are days when some medicines can be given while other
days should be avoided. It is also used to determine when to
harvest, process, and use plants as therapy. In addition to the
powers brought by each season, other energies are brought by
planetary configurations, modifying, increasing, or eliminating
the power and effects of the plant. This is a concept somewhat
known in Europe. For example, it is known that some plants
create poisons, under specific astrological influences and conditions, although they are habitually inoffensive. Likewise, in
some conditions, some excellent medicines can be made from
plants that are normally venomous.

Jacques Haesaert elegantly described astrology as follows:
"Astrology involves observing what happens in the universe:
A person can understand what is happening inside himself at
the same moment, according to the laws of correspondence.
Observation and knowledge of these laws even enable him
to anticipate the next movement and know what is going to
happen, since all movements follow certain laws. At the same
time, man possesses the potential to influence all movement
around him, through his divine creative power. In fact, he is
the cause of all movement."

CONCLUDING REMARKS

Tibetan medicine embodies many elements of medicine completely ignored—and in most cases unknown—to Western science, medicine, and society as a whole. Accepting some of the concepts of the Tibetan and other traditional medical systems is challenging, because the theories and practices first appear incomprehensible, especially due to their intangible and unquantifiable components.

Tibetan medicine is sometimes considered to be a kind of "alternative medicine", which tend to require the support of Western medicine in serious acute cases. Be that as it may, for many health problems, Tibetan medicine is as powerful as modern medicine and incurs significantly fewer side effects.

It is my hope that you now have a feeling for what this comprehensive medical tradition has to offer. Over many centuries, this integrative medical system has proven to be not only extremely effective but also complementary to modern Western medicine. While the latter excels in treating acute disorders, surgical procedures, diagnostic technology, and computer analyses, Tibetan medicine particularly excels in the treatment of chronic conditions. It also offers very precise diagnostic methods especially useful for disorders in babies and children, and valuable information about prevention and treatment.

Although much of the material in this book may have been alien to you at first acquaintance, hopefully you can take away useful insights that will promote your wellness and assist you in treating illness. If we are mindful of how our actions affect our health, we can live better, happier, healthier lives. We will want to avoid excesses, opt for the "middle road" of appropriate behavior and nutrition, and understand the importance of feeling satisfaction and appreciation of what we have. At the same time, we will want to work on eliminating our negative emotions, in order to develop positive feelings surrounding all that we do and thus find lasting happiness by developing compassion and directing it towards helping others.

Having a better idea of how to live harmoniously with nature, we can benefit from all that it has to offer—and understand that it provides us with exactly what we need! As nature is continuously undergoing changes, we must change with it, adapting to the seasons, climate, weather, our age, and so on, and do what is best for us at the time.

We can enjoy the great benefits of discarding our certitudes and accepting that there exists this imperceptible world of subtle energies that operates in our bodies, and opening our minds to how it explains many things that modern science is unable to. Becoming conscious of the countless invisible and visible beings surrounding us, we develop an awareness that we are all connected. Moreover, by realizing that we have responsibility for what happens to us, we can stop blaming others! In doing so, we stop wasting our time on trivia, negativity, and judgment and are given greater perspective in the face of difficulty.

Living in the present moment and developing openness to listen and benefit from ancient wisdom, with a readiness to change our preconceived ideas, will offer us benefits beyond what we could even imagine!

Components of the tree of medicine

3 roots, 9 trunks, 47 branches, 224 leaves (in italics)

Root 1. The human organism and functioning

Trunk 1. The healthy body: anatomy—physiology

Branch 1. The subtle energies—disorders
Sokzin lung (maintaining life), *kyengyu lung* (ascendant), *kyabche lung* (omni-penetrating), *menyam lung* (metabolic), and *thursel lung* (descendent), *juche triba* (digestive), *danggyur triba* (color-transforming), *drubche triba* (accomplishing), *thongche triba* (responsable for vision), and *doksel triba* (complexion-clearing), *tenche pegen* (supporting), *nyagche pegen* (mixing,) *nyongche pegen* (experiencing), *chorche pegen* (connecting), and *tshimche pegen* (satisfying)

Branch 2. The seven bodily constituents
Chyle, blood, flesh, fat, bone, bone marrow, regenerative substances
Flowers: health/purity/brilliance, long life
Fruits: dharma, wealth, happiness

Branch 3. The impurities
Excrement, urine, sweat

Trunk 2. State of imbalance: the diseased body

Branch 1. Primary causes
Attachment – *lung*; hatred – *triba*; ignorance – *pegen*

Branch 2. Secondary causes
Time—seasonal change, demonic influences, nutrition, behavior

Branch 3. Ways illnesses enter
Enter through pores of the skin, expand in the flesh, move through nerves, fix to bone, descend the solid organs, accumulate in the hollow organs

Branch 4. Main location of the energies
Upper region of the body – head – *pegen*
Middle region of the body – liver – *triba*
Lower region of the body – hips – *lung*

Branch 5. Passageways of the energies
Lung: bone, ears, hair—sense organs, heart, colon
Triba: blood, eyes, sweat, liver, intestines
Pegen: other corporal constituents, nose, tongue, excrement, urine, lungs, spleen, stomach, kidneys

Branch 6. Time of arising
Age:
elderly – *lung*; adult – *triba*; child – *pegen*
Place:
cold, wind – *lung*; dry and hot – *triba*; humid and oily – *pegen*
Time, season:
summer and sunset – *lung*; autumn, midday, and midnight – *triba*;
spring, morning and evening – *pegen*

Branch 7. Fatal disorders, results of karma
Merit used up, conjunction of cold and hot disorders, absence of treatment, worsening in spite of treatment, lesion

in vital organ by wounding, *lung* disorder too advanced, fever too advanced, cold disorder too advanced, corporal constituents intolerant of treatment, severe affliction caused by spirits

Branch 8. Imbalance of energies due to improper treatment
Lung healed, *triba* increased, *lung* healed, *pegen* increased; *lung* not healed, *triba* increased; *lung* not healed, *pegen* increased; *triba* healed, *lung* increased; *triba* healed, *pegen* increased; *triba* not healed, *lung* increased; *triba* not healed, *pegen* increased; *pegen* healed, *lung* increased; *pegen* healed, *triba* increased; *pegen* not healed, *lung* increased; *pegen* not healed, *triba* increased

Branch 9. Comparisons, affinities
Cold disorders – *lung* – cold, water
Hot disorders – blood – bile, heat, fire

Root 2. Diagnosis

Trunk 3. Visual observation methods

Branch 1. Tongue
Dry, red rough – *lung*; thick film, yellow – *triba*; light white film, humid – *pegen*

Branch 2. Urine
Blue, many bubbles – *lung*; strong smell, bubbles, a lot of vapor – *triba*; clear, no odor, little vapor – *pegen*

Trunk 4. Examination by touch

Branch 3. *Lung* pulse
Empty, large, intermittent

Branch 4. *Triba* pulse
rapid, full, taut

Branch 5. *Pegen* pulse
deep, weak, slow

Trunk 5. Methods of interrogation

Branch 6. Secondary causes/symptoms of *lung* disorders
Excessive light food, yawning, desire to stretch, chills, pain
in the joints, hips, kidneys, pain difficult to localize, changing, desire to vomit, problems of sight, protruding eyes,
intellectual weakness, symptoms more evident while fasting, improvement with rich, oily food

Branch 7. Secondary causes/symptoms of *triba* disorders
spicy hot, acrid food, excess heat in muscles, sharp pain in
upper body, bitter taste in the mouth, headache, symptoms
more obvious during digestion, refreshment gives relief

Branch 8. Secondary causes/symptoms of *pegen* disorders
excess oily, heavy food, loss of appetite, indigestion, repeated
vomiting, pasty mouth, stomach cramps, repeated belching,
mental and physical heaviness, feeling cold inside and outside, symptoms more evident after eating, relief with warm
food, clothing

Root 3. Treatment

Trunk 6. Nutrition

Branch 1. Foods suited for treating *lung*
Horse meat, donkey meat, groundhog meat, old dry meat,
human flesh, oil of seeds, old butter (> 1-year -old), old
brown sugar, garlic, onions

Branch 2. Drink suited for treating *lung*
Fresh warm milk, beer from barley with roots *(chava, ranie)*,
alcohol from brown sugar, alcohol from bones

Branch 3. Foods suited for treating *triba*
Cow or goat yogurt, whey, fresh butter, game, fresh meat of herbivores, fresh barley flour, a kind of spinach, a kind of dandelion

Branch 4. Drink suited for treating *triba*
Black tea, mineral water, melted snow, cooled boiled water

Branch 5. Foods suited for treating *pegen*
Mutton, wild yak, meat of carnivores, fish, honey, grilled barley flour, yak yogurt or whey

Branch 6. Drink suited for treating *pegen*
Old, strong, thick beer, hot boiled water

Trunk 7. Behavior

Branch 7. Behavior beneficial for *lung* disorders
Remain in warm place, be in company of pleasant friends

Branch 8. Behavior beneficial for *triba* disorders
Remain in cool place, act calmly

Branch 9. Behavior beneficial for *pegen* disorders
Warmth, activity

Trunk 8. Medication

Taste and medicinal qualities:
Branch 10. Tastes beneficial for *lung* disorders
Wweet (brown sugar), sour, salty

Branch 11. Qualities beneficial for *lung* disorders
Oily, heavy, soft

Branch 12. Tastes beneficial for *triba* disorders
Wweet, bitter, astringent

Branch 13. Qualities beneficial for *triba* disorders
Refreshing, light (not thick), softening

Branch 14. Tastes beneficial for *pegen* disorders
Acrid, spicy hot, sour, astringent

Branch 15. Qualities beneficial for *pegen* disorders
Acrid (like ammonia), rough, light
Different medicinal preparations:

Branch 16. Broths beneficial for *lung* disorders
Bone broth, meat broth + brown sugar + goat meat + beer +
butter + salt, old, dried sheep's head broth

Branch 17. Unctuous substances beneficial for *lung* disorders
Oil + nutmeg, oil + garlic, oil with five roots (*Rania, Tsawa,
Nye-shing, Asho, Sema*)
Oil with 3 fruits (*Terminalia chebula, Crataegus sanguinea, Cra-
taegus pinnatififa*)
Oil with poison (*sman-chen*)

Branch 18. Concoctions beneficial for *triba* disorders
Manu = *Bryonia, Tinospora cordifolia*, gentian, three fruits
(*Terminalia chebula, Crataegus sanguinea, Crataegus pinnatififa*)

Branch 19. Powders beneficial for *triba* disorders
Camphor, santal, saffron, bamboo manna

Branch 20. Pills beneficial for *pegen* disorders
Tsen-dug (anconitum, a poison), pills containing different
salts

Branch 21. Powders beneficial for *pegen*
Pomegranate, rhododendron, *Gö-ma-kha, lime mineral powder*,
burnt salts (*tchong-chi*)
Preparations with cleansing effects:

Branch 22. Enemas for *lung* disorders
Enema put in the end of colon, enema put farther up colon, *Tru-malen* enema

Branch 23. Purgation for *triba* disorders
Medicine preparing for purgation, direct purgative methods, rough methods, gentle methods

Branch 24. Induction of vomiting for *pegen* disorders – elimination
Gentle method, rough method

Trunk 9. External therapy

Branch 25. Treatments for *lung* disorders
Ointments with sesame oil
Envelopment with cloth saturated with hot cumin oil + butter + salt

Branch 26. Treatments for *triba* disorders
Induction of sweating, blood-letting, sitting under moving cold water

Branch 27. Treatments for *pegen* disorders
Envelopment with cloth saturated with hot boiled water, cauterization/moxa

REFERENCES

Anand, P., Kunnumakkara, A., Sundaram, C., Harikumar, K., Tharakan, S., Lai, O., Sung, B. and Aggarwal, B., 2008. Cancer is a Preventable Disease that Requires Major Lifestyle Changes. *Pharmaceutical Research*, 25(9), pp. 2200–2200.

Ba, D., Ssentongo, P., Beelman, R., Muscat, J., Gao, X. and Richie, J., 2021. Higher Mushroom Consumption is Associated with Lower Risk of Cancer: A Systematic Review and Meta-Analysis of Observational Studies. *Advances in Nutrition*, 12(5), pp. 1691–1704.

Bauer-Wu, S., Lhundup, T., Tidwell, T., Lhadon, T., Ozawa-de Silva, C., Dolma, J., Dorjee, P., Neshar, D., Sangmo, R. and Yeshi, T., 2014. Tibetan Medicine for Cancer. *Integrative Cancer Therapies*, 13(6), pp. 502–512.

Broadhead, G., Grigg, J., McCluskey, P., Hong, T., Schlub, T. and Chang, A., 2018. Saffron Therapy for the Treatment of Mild/ Moderate Age-Related Macular Degeneration: A Randomised Clinical Trial. *Graefe's Archive for Clinical and Experimental Ophthalmology*, 257(1), pp. 31–40.

CA: A Cancer Journal for Clinicians, 1996. Guidelines on Diet, Nutrition, and Cancer Prevention: Reducing the Risk of Cancer with Healthy Food Choices and Physical Activity. The American Cancer Society 1996 Advisory Committee on Diet, Nutrition, and Cancer Prevention, 46(6), pp. 325–341.

Coles, W., 1656. *The Art of Simpling: an Introduction to the Knowledge and Gathering of Plants*, Printed by J.G. for Nath. Brook.

143

Engel, S. and Tholstrup, T., 2015. Butter Increased Total and LDL Cholesterol Compared with Olive Oil but Resulted in Higher HDL Cholesterol Compared with a Habitual Diet. *The American Journal of Clinical Nutrition*, 102(2), pp. 309–315.

Kim, H., Yokoyama, W. and Davis, P., 2014. TRAMP Prostate Tumor Growth is Slowed by Walnut Diets Through Altered IGF-1 Levels, Energy Pathways, and Cholesterol Metabolism. *Journal of Medicinal Food*, 17(12), pp. 1281–1286.

Otsuki, N., Dang, N., Kumagai, E., Kondo, A., Iwata, S. and Morimoto, C., 2010. Aqueous Extract of Carica Papaya Leaves Exhibits Anti-Tumor Activity and Immunomodulatory Effects. *Journal of Ethnopharmacology*, 127(3), pp. 760–767.

Poulose, S., Miller, M. and Shukitt-Hale, B., 2014. Role of Walnuts in Maintaining Brain Health with Age. *The Journal of Nutrition*, 144(4), pp. 561S–566S.

Ramírez, J., Salazar, J., Fernández-Albarral, J., de Hoz, R., Ramírez, A., López-Cuenca, I., Salobrar-García, E. and Pinazo-Durán, M., 2020. Beneficial Effects of Saffron (Crocus sativus L.) in Ocular Pathologies, Particularly Neurodegenerative Retinal Diseases. *Neural Regeneration Research*, 15(8), p. 1408.

Sender, R., Fuchs, S. and Milo, R., 2016. Revised Estimates for the Number of Human and Bacteria Cells in the Body. *PLOS Biology*, 14(8), p. e1002533.

Shanafelt, T., Call, T., Zent, C., Leis, J., LaPlant, B., Bowen, D., Roos, M., Laumann, K., Ghosh, A., Lesnick, C., Lee, M., Yang, C., Jelinek, D., Erlichman, C. and Kay, N., 2012. Phase 2 Trial of Daily, Oral Polyphenon E in Patients with Asymptomatic, Rai Stage 0 To II Chronic Lymphocytic Leukemia. *Cancer*, 119(2), pp. 363–370.

Sharma, P., McClees, S. and Afaq, F., 2017. Pomegranate for Prevention and Treatment of Cancer: An Update. *Molecules*, 22(1), p. 177.

Thomas, J., 2009. Diet, Micronutrients, and the Prostate Gland. *Nutrition Reviews*, 57(4), pp. 95–103.

Zhang, Y., Talalay, P., Cho, C. and Posner, G., 1992. A Major Inducer of Anticarcinogenic Protective Enzymes from Broccoli: Isolation and Elucidation of Structure. *Proceedings of the National Academy of Sciences*, 89(6), pp. 2399–2403.

SUGGESTED READING

- *A Plea for the Animals: The Moral Philosophy and Evolutionary imperative to treat all beings with compassion*, by Matthieu Richard (2017) Shambhala Publications.
- *A Practical and Inspirational Guide to Diagnosing, Treating and Healing the Buddhist Way*, by Gerti Samel (2001) Little, Brown and Co.
- *Boundless healing, meditation exercises to enlighten the mind and heal the body*, by Tulku Thondrup Rinpoche (2000) Shambhala Publications.
- *China's Tibetan Medicine*, by Zhen Yan and Cai Jingfeng. (2005) Foreign language press.
- *Conquering Chronic Disease Through Vedic Medicine: The Complete Approach in Treating Chronic Complaints Without Side Effects*, by Kumuda Reddy and Linda Egenes (2002) New Age books.
- *Daring Steps: Traversing the Path of the Buddha*, by Ringu Tulku (2010) Edited and translated by Rosemarie Fuchs, published by Snow Lion Publications.
- *Health Through Balance*, by Dr. Yeshi Dhonden (1986) Snow Lion Publications.
- *Healthy Child and Mother, Happy Family*, by Dr. Lobsang Shrestha, in preparation.
- *Healing From the Source: The Science and Lore of Tibetan Medicine*, by Dr. Yeshi Dhonden (2000) Snow Lion Publications.

- *Remedies of energy and the universe*, by Dr. Jacques Echard. translated from French by Marilyn Magazin, in preparation.
- *Molecules of Emotions: The Science Behind Mind-Body Medicine*, by Candace B. Pert (1999) Simon and Schuster.
- *Studies in Tibetan Medicine*, by Finckh, Elisabeth, D.M. (1988) Snow Lion Publications.
- *The Art of Happiness*, by H.H. The Dalai Lama and Howard C. Cutler (1998) G.P. Putnam's Sons.
- *The Book of Tibetan Medicine: How to Use Tibetan Healing for Personal Well-being*, by Ralph Quinlan Forde (2008), Hachette Livre.
- *The Tibetan Book of Living and Dying*, by Sogyal Rinpoche (1992) Harper.
- *The Tibetan Book of Healing*, by Dr. Lopsang Rapgay, Ph.D. (1966) Pilgrims Publishers.
- The Tibetan Book of Health: *Sowa Rigpa*, the Science of Healing, by Nida Chenagtsang (2017) SKY Press.
- *The Tibetan Yogas of Dream and Sleep*, by Tenzin Wangyal Rinpoche (1998) Mark Dahlby, editor.
- *Tibetan Ayurveda: Health Secrets from the Roof of the World*, by Robert Sachs (1995) Healing Arts Press.
- *Tibetan Buddhist Medicine and Psychology: The Diamond Healing*, by Terry Clifford (1984) Motilal Banarsidass Publishers.
- *Tibetan Medicine and Other Holistic Health-care Systems*, by Tom Dumer (1988) Paljor Publications.
- *Tibetan Medicine: Illustrated in Original Texts*, by Rechung Rinpoche Jampal Kunzang (1973) University of California Press.
- *Tibetan Medicine—Medicine of Light: Teachings of Jacque Haesaert*, by the Association Ambroisie. Translated from French by Marilyn Magazin, in preparation.
- *Tibetan Medicine: The Buddhist Way of Healing*, by Dolkar Khangkar (1998) Roli Books Pvt Ltd.

INDEX

acupuncture, 103. *See also* therapy
alcoholism, 124
allergies, 119
Ambrosia Essence Tantra, 1
American diet, 59
anatomy, 17. *See also* physiology;
    psychology
    chakras, 33
    channels, 32, 34
    circulatory system, 32
    conception, 35
    dang, 36
    digestive system, 35
    elements of, 18, 32–40
    fear of death, 40
    five aggregates, 38
    mind and consciousness, 39
    organs, 37
    phantom pain, 37
    prana, 36
    seven bodily constituents, 36
    seven extractions, 36
anger, 22. *See also* three mental
    poisons
arthritis, 127–128
arthrosis, 127

art of palpation, 91. *See also*
    symptoms and diagnosis
asthma, 119–120
astringent plants, 113
astrological diagnosis, 97. *See also*
    symptoms and diagnosis
astrology, 131–132
awareness and mindfulness of
    moment, 51. *See also*
    behavior and nutrition

baby's sex determination, 45.
    See also conception
bardo, 42. *See also* conception
behavior, 139
behavior and nutrition, 51
    according to season, 52–57
    to avoid ill health, 58
    awareness and mindfulness of
    moment, 51
    body and the tree of life, 55–56
    cold food, 68
    consumption of drinks, 63
    diets and fasting, 78–79
    digestive fire, 54
    and disease, 57

du-chi, 65
eating according to seasons,
        75–76
food choices, 60
foods adapted to individual's
        needs, 59–65
foods for three dominant
        energy types, 65–68
foods to rectify energy
        imbalance, 67–68
"like heals like", 56–57
hot disorders, 65–66
maintaining health, 51
meditating, 63
overeating, 63
over-stimulating activities, 58
qualities and classification of
        food, 68–75
seasonal cycle of energies, 55
seasonal rhythms, 54
sex, 63
soy milk, 61
Tai Chi Chuan, 57
timing, 52
toxic foods and bad
        combinations, 77–78
weather conditions, 62–63
birth process, 46–47. *See also*
        childbirth
blood-letting, 104. *See also* therapy
bodhicitta, 2
body
    healthy, 135
    swelling, 128
body formation, 41, 45–46. *See also*
        childbirth; conception
    five elements, 42
    reincarnation and, 43
Buddhist concepts, 9
    consciousness, 14
    emptiness, 14

five aggregates, 15
    goal of Buddhist, 11
    goals in life, 9
    impermanence, 13–14
    karma in health and disease,
        11–12
    karmic connection between
        physician and patient, 12
    kind heart and unbiased
        compassion, 9–10
    mindfulness, 12–13
    mutual respect and
        confidence, 9
    physician's morality and
        motivation, 12
    samsara, 10–11
    three mental poisons, 14
    vital force, 15

cancer, 120–121
cardiac diseases, 121
cataracts, 121–122
chakras, 33
    and channels, 34
channels, 32, 34
childbirth, 41. *See also* body
        formation; conception
    health, 46–47
circulatory system, 32
cleansing, 114. *See also* therapy
cold food, 68. *See also* foods
cold or hot baths, 104. *See also*
        therapy
common cold, 122
conception, 35, 41–43. *See also*
        body formation;
        childbirth
    bardo, 42
    conditions for, 44–45
    consciousness's sokzin
        lung, 42

defective womb, 44
defects of *egg*, 44
determination of baby's sex, 45
karma, 41–42
reincarnation, 42
sperm-blood mixture, 41
subtle energy of desire, 42
consciousness, 14. *See also*
        Buddhist concepts;
        conception
    sokzin lung, 4
consultations, 91. *See also*
        symptoms and diagnosis
consumption of drinks, 63. *See also*
        behavior and nutrition
conventional truth, 20. *See also*
        three mental poisons
corn syrup, high fructose, 126
cupping, 104. *See also* therapy

dang, 36
decoctions, 114. *See also* therapy
defective womb, 44. *See also*
        conception
demons, 87. *See also* invisible
        powers and spirits
depression, 122–123
desire, 21–22. *See also* three mental
        poisons
dharma, 3
diabetes, 123
diagnosis, 93, 137–138. *See also*
        symptoms and diagnosis
diagnostic techniques, 90. *See also*
        symptoms and diagnosis
diarrhea, 123–124
diets, 78–79, 107–108. *See also*
        foods; therapy
digestive fire, 54
digestive system, 35
disease, 58, 81, 117–118

behavior and, 57
causes and conditions for
        diseases manifestation,
        82
characteristics of, 82
classes of, 83–84
fevers, 84
negative emotion to, 24–25
teachings on, 81
wounds, 84
disorder, 81–83. *See also* disease
doctrine of similarity, 112–113.
        See also therapy
dominant energy
    characteristics influenced by,
        31–32
    foods for, 65–68
dreams, 129–130
drug addiction, 124
du-chi, 65

eating according to seasons, 75–76.
        See also behavior and
        nutrition
egg defects, 44. *See also*
        conception
ego, 23. *See also* three mental
        poisons
emotions, 25. *See also* three mental
        poisons
emptiness, 14. *See also* Buddhist
        concepts
energy, 25. *See also* Buddhist
        concepts; three subtle
        energies
    of planes, 10
    seasonal cycle of, 55
epilepsy, 124–125
essential oils, 103. *See also*
        therapy
examination by touch, 137–138

fasting, 78–79. *See also* foods
fear of death, 40
fevers, 84. *See also* disease
fire, digestive, 54
five aggregates, 15, 38. *See also*
        Buddhist concepts
five elements, 19
    formation of body, 42
foods. *See also* behavior and
        nutrition
    adapted to individual's needs,
        59–65
    choices, 60
    cold, 68
    for dominant energy types,
        65–68
    eating according to seasons,
        75–76
    fruits, 72–73
    grains, 69–70
    groups, 69
    liquids, 73–75
    meats, 71
    oils, 70–71
    qualities and classification of,
        68–75
    recommended for energy
        imbalance, 67–68
    and season, 76
    toxic and bad combinations,
        77–78
    vegetables, 71–72
fructose corn syrup, high, 126
fruits, 72–73
    with hairs, 121

ghosts, hungry, 87. *See also*
        invisible powers and
        spirits
Gyü Shi, 17

Haesaert, J., xix, 11, 29, 38, 42, 86,
        101, 117, 132
hatred, 22. *See also* three mental
        poisons
healing, 99
    spiritual, 100
health, 49
    balance of energies, 49
    karma, 49–50
    maintaining health, 51
healthy body, 135
herbal medicine, 102. *See also*
        therapy
holistic medicine, 2
hot disorders, 65–66
hot-tasting spices, 75. *See also*
        foods
human organism and functioning,
        135–137
humors. *See* subtle energy
hungry ghosts, 87. *See also* invisible
        powers and spirits
hypertension, 125

ignorance, 20–21. *See also* three
        mental poisons
internal vital principles. *See* subtle
        energy
interrogation methods, 138
intuition. *See* signs
invisible powers and spirits, 85
    causes of reincarnation, 88
    demons, 87
    harmful spirits, 87
    hungry ghosts, 87
    narak, 87–88
    possession, 86
    in religion, 85
    sadak guardians, 86, 88
    spirit realm, 86

karma, 11–12, 41–42. *See also* Buddhist concepts; conception

"like heals like", 56–57. *See also* behavior and nutrition
lung. See also symptoms and diagnosis; three subtle energies
    disorders, 89, 115, 122
    energy, 27, 35, 37
    types, 27–28

mantras, 2
massage, 103–104. *See also* therapy
medication, 139–141
medicinal plant harvesting, 114. *See also* therapy
medicinal powders, 114. *See also* therapy
medicine
    herbal, 102. *See also* therapy
    holistic, 2
meditating, 63
menstrual disorders, 125
mind
    and consciousness, 39
    in disease, 106
mindfulness, 12–13. *See also* Buddhist concepts
mineral baths, 104. *See also* therapy
moxabustion, 103. *See also* therapy

narak, 87–88. *See also* invisible powers and spirits
negative emotion to disease, 24–25. *See also* three mental poisons

nutrition, 108–111, 138–139. *See also* therapy

obesity, 126
observation and questioning, 90–97. *See also* symptoms and diagnosis
omens, 129–130
organs, 37
overeating, 63. *See also* behavior and nutrition
over-stimulating activities, 58. *See also* behavior and nutrition

pacification, 114. *See also* therapy
Paracelsus, 56, 112
paralysis, 126–127
parasitic diseases, 127
patient-physician dialogue, 91. *See also* symptoms and diagnosis
pegen. See also symptoms and diagnosis; three subtle energies
    disorders, 90, 115
    energy, 28–29, 35–37
    types, 29
person's energy type, 30
    characteristics influenced by dominant energies, 31–32
    person's heredity, 31
phantom pain, 37
physiology, 17–18. *See also* anatomy; psychology
    chakras, 33
    channels, 32, 34
    circulatory system, 32
    conception, 35
    dang, 36

digestive system, 35
elements of anatomy and, 32–40
fear of death, 40
five aggregates, 38
mind and consciousness, 39
organs, 37
phantom pain, 37
prana, 36
seven bodily constituents, 36
seven extractions, 36
prana, 36
pregnant woman, 46–47. *See also* childbirth
protective foods, 110
psychology, 17. *See also* anatomy; physiology; three mental poisons

"realms" of existence, 10. *See also* Buddhist concepts
reincarnation, 10, 42. *See also* Buddhist concepts; conception
and body formation, 43
rheumatism, 127–128
rheumatoid arthritis, 127
rhythms, 18

sadak guardians, 86, 88. *See also* invisible powers and spirits
samsara, 10–11. *See also* Buddhist concepts
seasonal
cycle of energies, 55
rhythms, 54
seven bodily constituents, 36
seven extractions, 36
sex, 63
Shrestha, L., xx, 62, 120

signs, 129–130
similarity, doctrine of, 112–113. *See also* therapy
soy milk, 61. *See also* foods
sperm-blood mixture, 41. *See also* conception
spirit, 87, 97. *See also* invisible powers and spirits; symptoms and diagnosis
detection, 97
realm, 86
state of imbalance, 136–137
stevia, 60
subtle energy, 25. *See also* three subtle energies
of desire, 42
swelling, 128
symptoms and diagnosis, 89
art of palpation, 91
astrological diagnosis and detection of spirits, 97
color of veins, 95–96
consultations, 91
correspondence of zones of ears and organs, 95
diagnosis, 93
diagnostic techniques, 90
ear observation, 96
lung disorders, 89
maternal milk observation, 94
observation, 92–97
observation and questioning, 90
patient-physician dialogue, 91
pegen disorders, 90
spirits, 97
symptoms, 89–90
taking of pulse, 91–92
triba disorder, 90
urine analysis, 92–93

Tai Chi Chuan, 57, 128
taking of pulse, 91–92. *See also*
     symptoms and diagnosis
tantra, 24
therapy, 101
    acupuncture, 103
    adjusting one's behavior,
      106–107
    blood-letting, 104
    categories of treatment, 101
    cold or hot baths, 104
    cupping, 104
    decoctions, 114
    diet as therapy, 107–108
    doctrine of similarity, 112–113
    essential oils, 103
    external, 141
    harvesting of medicinal plants,
      114
    herbal medicine, 102
    ingredients of medicinal
      powders, 114
    lung disorders, 115
    massage, 103–104
    medicines and other
      treatments, 111–115
    mineral baths, 104
    moxabustion, 103
    nutrition as therapy, 108–111
    pacification and cleansing, 114
    pegen disorders, 115
    protective foods, 110
    role of mind in disease, 106
    for sick baby, 107
    treatments, 102–107
    triba disorders, 115
The Tree of Life, 55
    body and, 55–56
    "like heals like", 56
the tree of medicine
    behavior, 139
    components of, 135
    diagnosis, 137–138
    examination by touch, 137–138
    external therapy, 141
    healthy body, 135
    human organism and
      functioning, 135–137
    medication, 139–141
    methods of interrogation, 138
    nutrition, 138–139
    state of imbalance, 136–137
    treatment, 138–141
    visual observation methods,
      137
three mental poisons, 14, 19. *See
    also* Buddhist concepts
    anger and hatred, 22
    conventional truth, 20
    desire, 21–22
    ego, 23
    emotions, 25
    ignorance, 20–21
    negative emotion to disease,
      24–25
    ultimate truth, 20
three subtle energies, 25–26, 35–37.
    See also subtle energy
    balance of, 49
    energy, 25
    health and disease, 25
    lung energy, 27, 35, 37
    lung types, 27–28
    pegen energy, 28–29, 35–37
    pegen types, 29
    physiological functions and,
      27–29
    and principal paths, 30
    source, 27
    triba energy, 28, 35, 37
    triba types, 28
thursel lung, 125

Tibet, xvii
Tibetan doctor, xvii, 7, 61
    becoming a, 3
Tibetan medicine, xvii, xix, 1–7, 83,
        101, 133. *See also* Tibetan
        Medicine Tree
    allergies, 119
    Ambrosia Essence Tantra, 1
    anatomy, physiology, and
        psychology, 17
    asthma, 119–120
    bodhicitta, 2
    cancer, 120–121
    cardiac diseases, 121
    cataracts, 121–122
    common cold, 122
    components, 111
    depression, 122–123
    diabetes, 123
    diarrhea, 123–124
    to diseases, 119
    drug addiction and
        alcoholism, 124
    epilepsy, 124–125
    fundamental aspects of, 1
    hypertension, 125
    mantras, 2
    menstrual disorders, 125
    obesity, 126
    paralysis, 126–127
    parasitic diseases, 127
    rheumatism and arthritis,
        127–128
    swelling of body, 128

thursel lung, 125
    Western dogmas absent from,
        117–118
Tibetan Medicine Tree, 3
    prime feature of, 5
    root one, 3–4
    root three, 4, 6
    root two, 4–5
toxic foods, 77–78. *See also* foods
treatment, 138–141
triba. See also symptoms and
        diagnosis; three subtle
        energies
    disorder, 90, 115
    energy, 28, 35, 37
    types, 28

ultimate truth, 20. *See also* three
        mental poisons
urine analysis, 92–93. *See also*
        symptoms and diagnosis

Vajrayāna, 24
vaporising essential oils, 58
verbena (*Verveine officinale*), 113
visual observation methods, 137
vital force, 15. *See also* Buddhist
        concepts
vital points, 18

weather conditions, 62–63
wounds, 84. *See also* disease